Sandra Rabello de Frias

Institutionalising Old People

Sandra Rabello de Frias

Institutionalising Old People

A space for reminiscence and resistance

ScienciaScripts

Imprint

Cover image: www.ingimage.com

This book is a translation from the original published under ISBN 978-613-9-67792-4.

Publisher:
Sciencia Scripts
is a trademark of
Dodo Books Indian Ocean Ltd. and OmniScriptum S.R.L publishing group

120 High Road, East Finchley, London, N2 9ED, United Kingdom
Str. Armeneasca 28/1, office 1, Chisinau MD-2012, Republic of Moldova, Europe
Printed at: see last page
ISBN: 978-620-7-70061-5

Eros is the most beautiful, and I hasten to tell you why: first of all, dear Phaedrus, because he is the youngest of the gods, and of this quality he himself provides us with an obvious proof: that by running away, he avoids being caught up in old age, which is undeniably fast in itself, as I can see from the fact that he comes to us faster than he should.
Eros, in keeping with his own nature, truly hates old age and can't stand it, even at a great distance.

Agatao's speech
"The Banquet
PLATAO

ACKNOWLEDGMENTS

To God, in eternal gratitude.
To my husband Sandro for his encouragement, collaboration and understanding of my absences and time away.
To my mother, 'in memoria', for encouraging me to take up the cause of growing old.
To my cousin Cleonice, who told me on the phone one Sunday afternoon that everything would work out.

To my dear advisor Fatima who, with all her spirituality, helped me at various times during this journey, bringing security, knowledge and firmness to the construction of this work.
I would like to thank Professor Marcelo who, with his knowledge and academic practice, made me see further. To Professor Auterives, whose vast knowledge of philosophy and generosity gave me the air of a thinker.
To the teachers and staff of the Veiga de Almeida University Tijuca Campus for their support.
To my friend Roberto, my partner in the master's program, for the many academic conversations we had in order to win a battle.

UnATi for providing me with a great foundation for my professional and academic experience.
To the elderly people I've worked with over the last twenty-three years in Gerontology
Andreia, my professional and work colleague, for helping me with her excellent performance in organizing bibliographic standards.

And finally my little dog Mocinha, who has always been by my side, lying next to the computer waiting for us to be together again.

SUMMARY

This dissertation carried out a conceptual theoretical study on aging and the major changes that accompany this process in our society, emphasizing the implications for the institutionalization of the elderly. Based on considerations about the phenomenon of aging in Brazil, the research sought to analyze the context of old people's shelters and the care provided by Long Stay Institutions (ILPIs). Our general aim was to reflect on the socio-historical aspects that make up an institution for the care of the elderly and the repercussions of the process of institutionalization on aging and frail individuals. The specific objectives were: to describe the gerontological practices carried out in ILPIs and the nuances achieved by the perception of the ageing process; to problematize institutionalized old age in an interdisciplinary way; to present the psychoanalytical aspects that affect the discomfort of growing old in contemporary times; to research issues relating to enclosure, reminiscence and resistance. In order to uncover the institutional space of old people in greater depth, we used the notions of total institution, disciplinary power and cultural malaise, from Goffman, Foucault and Freud respectively, as our central concepts. Our methodology was to revisit the practices of confinement theoretically, using surrealist cinema to problematize the proposed theme. The result of this work examines, through a critical eye, the relations of power and care engendered by the institutionalization of the elderly, problematizing knowledge about institutions for the elderly, in order to propose an "ethic of existence", which needs to be embraced by care that gives space to desire, resist and remember.

Keywords: asylum, desire, care, old age

SUMMARY

1. INTRODUCTION

Are long-term care facilities for the elderly treating institutionalized people as subjects of desire and rights?

Thinking about aging and the great changes that accompany this process in our society, we saw the need to develop a theoretical and reflective research that would propose a conceptual outline of the socio-historical repercussions that involve aging (people in a process of physical and psychosocial fragility or with chronic illnesses) and its implications for institutionalization, as a means of ensuring global life care.

This paper aims to analyze the context of the institutionalization of old people and the care provided to the elderly by Long-Term Care Institutions (LTCIEs). Based on considerations about the phenomenon of ageing in Brazil, this work aims to uncover the care processes carried out by ILPIs, problematizing knowledge about institutions for the elderly, in order to propose an ethic of existence.

Our *object of study* is to reflect on the socio-historical aspects that make up an institution for the care of the elderly and the repercussions of the process of institutionalization on aging and frail subjects. We will carry out a theoretical study in the light of the three main thinkers, Goffman, Foucault and Freud, revisiting practices of confinement and making use of surrealist cinema as a problematizer of the proposed theme.

ILPIs, as they are called through the Social Assistance policy, are closed institutions with their own rules and specific legislation that accompanies their operation. ILPIs are characterized by physical locations 1 Social Assistance, established as a social right as part of the social security system in the Federal Constitution (1988), has the formative principles of providing free services and basically protecting the family, motherhood, childhood, adolescence and old age, as well as the disabled and reintegrating those who need it into the job market. "Social assistance is the autonomous segment of social security that deals with the underprivileged, i.e. those who are unable to provide for themselves. It takes care of those with the greatest needs, without requiring them (its beneficiaries) to make any contribution to social security" (BRASIL, 1988).

equipped to take care of people aged 60 or over, on a boarding basis, for a fee or not, for an indefinite period. These establishments usually have different denominations and human resources to meet the needs of the elderly in the areas of social assistance, health, food, hygiene, rest and leisure, as well as other activities to ensure quality of life.

In order to uncover the institutional space of old people in greater depth, we intend to delve into the universe of closed institutions, which GOFFMAN (2015) calls total institutions.

> When we review the different institutions of our Western society, we find that some are more "closed" than others. Their "closure" or total character is symbolized by the barrier to social intercourse with the outside world and by prohibitions to exit that are often included in the physical scheme - for example, closed doors, high walls, barbed wire, moats, water, forests or swamps (GOFFMAN, 2015, p.16).

The institutions that care for the elderly are still places to be discovered. These institutions were born in Brazil out of charitable efforts, intensified in the 19th century during Imperial Brazil, and since then, they have gained social prominence, with the intention of promoting hygienization in the social context of that time. In the field of the social history of asylums, our research will problematize the historical context, bringing in the facts, the social and political issues of the time when the first asylums were set up in Brazil and the impact of this asylums model that has reached the present day.

According to Goffman (2015),

> a total institution can be defined as a place of residence and work where a large number of similarly situated individuals, separated from the wider society for a considerable period of time, lead a closed and formally administered life (GOFFMAN, 2015, p.11).

In his research on the institutionalization of old people, Groisman (1999a) reflects on the effects of nursing homes on the institutionalized elderly. The author considers that the institutionalization of old age is a powerful mechanism for producing meanings and stigmas about the aging process, reinforcing the negative image of old age and the various processes through which the old subject experiences helplessness. The author points out that institutionalized old age ends up accelerating decrepitude, illness and disability, stressing that only in these closed spaces will the evils and ills characteristic of an old age in seclusion be allowed.

Reflecting on the historical processes of humanity, and looking at modernity, we can see apparent transformations in the structure of the world's population. Social, political and economic phenomena have characterized major conflicts in the world, such as wars and genocides, which have certainly had an impact on the world's demographics. Before the Industrial Revolution, the population had a low life expectancy and a high mortality rate. Countries like England had a strong impact on advances in medicine, scientific research aimed at pharmaceutical industrialization, the organization of cities for basic sanitation and the growing urbanization of large centers, where job opportunities favoured increased income and improved quality of life for those populations.

The *United Nations Population Division* (UN, 2015) points out that changes in fertility and mortality rates are related to economic and social transformations. The organization points to the reduction in infant mortality, improved access to education and employment opportunities, advances in gender equality, developments in reproductive health and the promotion of family planning as factors that have contributed to the reduction in the fertility rate. In addition, advances in public health and technologies associated with medicine, accompanied by improved housing conditions, mean that people live longer and healthier lives than before, particularly at older ages (SOUZA; MELO, 2017).

However, it should be emphasized that the factors that have led to a reduction in mortality rates have also led to an increase in life expectancy. For this reason, we can see that the world population is going through a process of epidemiological transition of great magnitude, characterized by longevity. Most countries have experienced an increase in the number of elderly people in their populations. The intense and growing ageing of the world's population, considering the data in the report published by the WHO (2015), says that between 2015 and 2030, the number of people over 60 is expected to grow by 56%, from 901 million to 1.4 billion, and that by 2050, the global population of elderly people is projected to more than double that of 2015, reaching around 2.1 billion.

When it comes to the *oldest-old, i.e. the* late elderly, people over the age of 80, the projection shows an even greater growth than the elderly in general, reaching 434 million in 2050, which is more than triple the 125 million observed in 2015.

The process that began more than a century ago in the more developed nations is currently proving to be more vigorous in the less developed nations, so that over the next 15 years, Latin America and the Caribbean are projected to see a 71% increase in the population aged over 60, followed by Asia (66%), Africa (64%), Oceania (57%), North America (41%) and Europe (23%) (SOUZA; MELO, 2017).

With all this effervescent scenario regarding the aging process in the country, we felt the need to deepen a theoretical, exploratory study with an analytical basis that would focus on the long-lived elderly who suffer the process of institutionalization.

The institutionalization of the elderly is essentially a process of long-term care. Long-term care consists of a set of activities of daily living (ADLs). This set of activities should follow a routine of procedures which, if well developed and well supervised, can promote the quality of life of those who need it. But long-term care is not just a sequence of procedures, because in order to carry out these activities perfectly, institutions that care for elderly people in the process of frailty must have a team that is well trained in care procedures and in meeting the various needs that an institutionalized elderly person has.

With regard to the impressions of the institution for sick, old and abandoned people, our research also intends to work with the universe of images and, to this end, we intend to use cinematographic language to translate the concerns pertinent to the object studied and the various social manifestations that lead aging individuals to be in an institution for the elderly in pure confinement. At this point, we will bring together concepts from sociological, historical and psychoanalytical analysis.

The asylum is basically a bureaucratic institution, whose hierarchy derives from the position that each person occupies within it. They establish relations of power that are expressions of an organization, which is characterized by rules and regulations which, as rational elements, represent the specialized knowledge of those who exercise their functions over the inmates. They are treated as objects over which the work of keeping them alive and reasonably comfortable is carried out, while death - its obvious, imminent and inevitable prospect - does not come to take them away for good. (SOUZA, 2003, p. 2).

The aging process, old age, loss, institutionalization strategies, total institutions, disciplinary tactics, ways of framing the self, forms of care and practices of the self are some of the concepts to be approached from a Freudian psychoanalytical perspective, from a sociological perspective according to Goffman and from a historical perspective in the light of Foucault. The aim is to identify how old people live with their desires, reminiscences and mechanisms of resistance in a closed space that demarcates routine and daily life in patterns of surveillance and control.

With regard to public policies, we could not fail to include them in this work, given the importance of legal instruments to ensure the fundamental rights and guarantees of the elderly in Brazil. The processes of regulating the human rights of the elderly will be detailed. It is necessary to reflect on the advances and small achievements that the Brazilian elderly have made since the promulgation of Law 8.842/94, regulated by Decree 1948/1996, known as the National Policy for the Elderly.

According to Hathaway (2017), in Brazil the protection of the elderly as a vulnerable group is guaranteed by the Constitution of the Republic (CR)[2] , in Chapter II, which deals with health as a "right of all and duty of the State" (art. 196).), especially by guaranteeing the welfare benefit of one minimum monthly wage to the elderly who can prove that they do not have the means to support themselves or have their family support them[3] (art.203,V), and in Chapter VII, which deals with the rights of the family, children, adolescents, young people and the elderly (arts.226 to 230).

The 1988 Constitution recognizes the family as the basis of society, which in turn deserves special protection from the state (art. 226). Paragraph 8 of art. 226 states that the state shall ensure assistance to the family in the person of each of its members, creating mechanisms to curb violence in their relations. The Constitution states that children have a duty to help support their parents in old age, need or

---

2 It was only in the 1988 Constitution "that social security, health and social assistance policies were reorganized and restructured with new principles and guidelines and became part of the Brazilian social security system" (BOSCHETTI, 2010, p. 8).

3 Specifically on the issue of the elderly and the formation of the social protection system after 1988, Teixeira (2007) emphasizes the importance of non-contributory benefits that do not follow the logic of insurance, especially the Continuous Cash Benefit (BPC), which provides assistance of 1 national minimum wage to the elderly who meet the eligibility criteria.

illness (Art. 229).

Article 230 of the Constitution of the Republic establishes that the family, society and the state have a duty to support the elderly, ensuring their participation in the community, defending their dignity and well-being and guaranteeing them the right to life. The Constitution also stipulates that programs to support the elderly should preferably be carried out in their homes (art. 230, para. 1), and grants the over-65s free urban public transport (art. 230, para. 2).

The constitutional design of fundamental rights in Brazil, focused on issues inherent to ageing, will be of great importance in building the legislative pillars that will underpin the narratives of this work.

In Chapter 1, we describe the gerontological practices carried out in ILPIs and the nuances achieved by the perception of the ageing process. There is a contextualization of some current developments in our country's public policy scene. Another important aspect of this chapter is the problematization of old age as a social category, as it has been conceptualized in the light of some aging scholars. Negotiations about the subject and desire in a time of loss are discussed, a theme illuminated by Freud's considerations.

In Chapter 2, we analyze the historical, political and social perspectives of institutionalized old age, contextualizing the birth of asylums in Brazil and situating the regulatory frameworks of public policies aimed at ILPIs. In the sociological and historical fields, it is essential to delve into the works of Goffman and Foucault. The focus of the study is to understand the strategies of mortification of the self in total institutions, as presented by Goffman. It also discusses the circumstances in which disciplinary powers affect bodies, leading to a framing of the self and the stripping away of its identity, a theme developed by Foucault. The notions of biopower and biopolitics conclude some of the reflections in this chapter, by discussing the health processes of an ageing population.

In Chapter 3, we deal with some psychoanalytic aspects in dialogue with issues related to ageing. Issues relating to the discomfort of ageing in contemporary times are discussed. There is a deepening of a Foucauldian reflection, based on the notions of disciplinary institutions and docile bodies and the modes of resistance that take into account certain care and practices of the self. The notion of social memory allows for a contextualization of the concept of reminiscence, situating it as another form of resistance, a term also understood in the Foucauldian sense. Institutionalized old age is finally considered from the point of view of the effects of confinement and the importance of reminiscence and resistance as guiding principles for an ethic of existence in ILPIs.

With this work, we hope to make a contribution to the scenario of long-term care institutions for the elderly in Brazil. Institutes and their elders must be much more than a form of care for the physically, cognitively, emotionally or socially fragile elderly; they must be open to contemporary innovations, allowing social behaviors, dreams and desires to come and go at the end of human life.

2. AGING AND CARE IN A TIME OF LOSS

In this chapter, we will reflect on population aging, presenting some conceptualizations of old age and various aspects that characterize the process of growing old, from normal old age to frail and institutionalized old age. The phenomenon of ageing has recently taken over academic circles, bringing up social issues that have not yet been debated, such as how individuals will face old age and its consequences, the impact of loss and the institutionalization of care in old age. After all, ageing has countless subjective, social and economic repercussions, encouraging the development of public policies and raising awareness of the growing demand for support for an ageing population.

In seeking to understand the subjective and social effects of growing old in a time of loss, in the light of some psychoanalytic concepts, we realize that reflecting on the aging process brings with it a natural restlessness about the anxieties, anxieties, dilemmas and possibilities that we will have to face about our own process of growing old.

2.1. Ageing and institutionalization: a space to be revisited

When we talk about human aging, it's worth noting that the aging process doesn't occur homogeneously for all individuals. It involves structural development factors in each country, as well as personal factors for each individual, such as lifestyle, genetic factors and psychosocial factors. Considering these international differences, the UN considers the onset of old age to be the age of 60 for developing countries and 65 for developed countries.

The ageing of the population has been of great concern to international organizations and some countries, which need to understand the various demographic aspects that have radically affected their demographic pyramid.

A UN study (2017) on the world population concluded that life expectancy has increased in all regions of the world, from 67.2 years in 2000-2005 to 70.8 years in 2010-2015. Population ageing in the world has seen an approximate 3% increase in the population aged over 60 every year. In 2017, it is estimated that the elderly will make up 13% of the general population, which represents around 962 million people over the age of 60. By 2050, this group is projected to represent 2.1 billion of the general population.

To draw a historical and contemporary parallel to the process of the world's ageing population, let's start with the First World General Assembly of the United Nations Organization, which convened the first World Meeting on Ageing in Vienna, Austria in 1982. This Assembly was attended by 125 countries, including Brazil. This Assembly approved the International Plan of Action on Ageing, which provided perspectives on plans, programs and policies that would strengthen the guidelines for a new world order on ageing, especially in developing countries.

Twenty years later, in April 2002, the second World Assembly on Ageing was held in Madrid (Spain), which approved a recommendation on investments in public policies, with the aim of implementing programs that would guarantee ageing populations support and investments that would promote longevity, dignity and quality of life for all individuals, especially those most in need of basic priorities, with a view to social inclusion and human dignity.

In this global panorama, considering some economic and historical aspects, it is worth noting that Brazil has been going through the aging process at a very fast pace. This accelerated process could influence the implementation of effective public policies to guarantee society the necessary conditions for ageing in terms of the various multifactorial aspects that determine the success of an ageing population.

Brazil is following the global trend and is aging, with some delay compared to developed countries. Data from the IBGE (2015) shows that the life expectancy of Brazilians rose from 45 years in 1940 to 75.5 years in 2015. This increase in life expectancy has had an impact on the percentage of elderly people in the total population. Checking the WHO's demographic statistics (2015), we see that the percentage of people over 60 in Brazil rose from 6.4% of the total population in 1990 to 11.7% in 2015.

The ageing of the population brings with it significant consequences in terms of demographic change and the need to implement public policies to assist the ageing population. Changes must take place primarily in the areas of health and social assistance, spreading care plans, self-care and a good extension of institutional and community support networks among the ageing population and their carers.

According to Lucchesi (2017), Brazil's population began a rapid process of aging due to the reduction in the fertility rate, which occurred in the mid-1960s, leading to an increase in the longevity of Brazilians. The total fertility rate fell from 6.28 children per woman in 1960 to 1.90 children in 2010 - a reduction of around 70%. In the same period, life expectancy at birth increased by 25 years, reaching 73.4 years in 2010 (IBGE, 2012, apud LUCCHESI, 2017).

According to Lucchesi (2017), the increase in life expectancy goes hand in hand with the decrease in the number of children per woman. The total fertility rate is currently 1.77 children on average per woman; by 2030, the forecast is that the rate will fall to 1.5. According to experts, the rate is already below that considered necessary for the natural replacement of the population, of 2.1 children per woman. The survey highlights that the drop in the number of children will be registered even in states that currently have rates above the national average, such as Acre (2.6 children per woman) or Amazonas (2.4 children per woman). There, the coefficient will fall to 1.8 children and 1.4 children per woman in 2030 respectively (IBGE, 2012).

According to Lucchesi (2017), the lower number of children, a trend since the 1970s, is also explained by the postponement of motherhood. In 2013, Brazilian women had their first child at the age of 26.9 on average. In 2030, they will have their first child almost three years later, at the age of 29.3. According to IBGE, the number of Brazilians will grow in geometric progression until 2042. (IBGE, 2012).

The aging of the population in Brazil poses important challenges for health care and social assistance, as well as for the institutional care network for the elderly. According to Camarano (2012), ageing is more than a risk to life, it represents a threat to an individual's autonomy and independence. Studies by the World Health Organization (WHO) in 1984 estimated that in a cutoff in which 75% of individuals survive to the age of 70, around 1/3 of them will have chronic illnesses, and at least 20% will have some degree of associated disability. This leads to immediate concern about the increase in demand for health services and the costs this entails (CAMARANO, 2012).

According to Lucchesi (2017), population ageing points to the prospect of the elderly being affected by degenerative and chronic diseases, which reduces or removes their autonomy, i.e. makes them dependent on someone else's care. Health studies (KARSCH, 1998; 2003, apud KUCHEMANN, 2012) indicate that, at the turn of the century, around 40% of people aged 65 and over needed some kind of help to carry out tasks such as shopping, looking after their finances, preparing meals and cleaning the house. A smaller proportion (10%) were considered to lack autonomy to carry out basic tasks such as bathing, dressing, going to the toilet, eating, sitting down and getting up from chairs and beds. The data indicates that activities involving care should gradually gain in importance in the aspects involving the degenerative processes of human ageing.

Some elderly people require institutionalization because they are old and highly dependent, because their family ties have broken down, because they have no family to build on, because they have been abandoned or because they have difficulty finding financial support. Long-stay institutions for the elderly (ILPIs) sometimes become necessary as a last resort to support the elderly.

Law 8.842, of January 4, 1994, which provides for the National Policy for the Elderly, regulated by Decree 1.948, of August 3, 1996, states in Article 3 that the asylums of social assistance for the elderly are understood to be the following

In the first paragraph of the article, it states that "in-home care is provided to elderly people who have no family ties or who are unable to provide for themselves, in order to meet their needs for housing, food, health and social interaction". The article's sole paragraph states that "nursing home care is provided in the event of the absence of a family group, abandonment, lack of financial resources or the family's own financial resources.

In our society, nursing homes play the role of guardians of the elderly who need them, without having to rethink new ways of protecting long-lived and frail individuals, with a view to improving the procedures and innovations that accompany contemporaneity. Asylums need to be re-conceptualized so that their function can be detached from old dogmas and outdated concepts, with a view to reconnecting with the new way of growing old.

The total institutions of our society can be *roughly* divided into five groups. Firstly, there are institutions set up to care for people who are thought to be incapable and harmless; these include homes for the blind, the old, orphans and the destitute (GOFFMAN, 2015, p.16).

Based on Goffman (2015), thinking of institutions as closed spaces, with disciplinary rules and without the promotion of guaranteeing the possibilities of those who occupy them, leads us to imagine in what perspectives aging subjects will be able to rework their lives after institutionalization.

> Secondly, there are places set up to look after people who are considered incapable of looking after themselves and who are also a threat to the community, albeit unintentionally; sanatoria for tuberculosis, hospitals for the mentally ill and leprosaria (GOFFMAN, 2015, p.16).

Contextualizing in Goffman (2015) the confinement spaces of people said to be incapable of taking care of themselves, we saw that the aspects that emerge between the subjects in the power relationship between those considered by the system to be stronger over the weaker predominate, imposing rules and routines on individuals with low esteem that are configured in practices and relationships of power over the supposedly weak.

> A third type of total institution is organized to protect the community from intentional dangers, and the well-being of the people thus isolated is not the immediate problem: jails, penitentiaries, prisoner of war camps, concentration camps (GOFFMAN, 2015, p.16).

In this paragraph, Goffman (2015) defines what he considers to be the framework that will determine those who are in the process of imprisonment to follow the norms for good behavior chosen by institutional power relations.

> Fourthly, there are institutions established with the intention of carrying out some work task more adequately, and which are justified only by such instrumental foundations: barracks, ships, boarding schools, labor camps, colonies and large mansions (from the point of view of those who live in servants' housing). (GOFFMAN, 2015, p.16).

Norms and disciplinary rules are characteristics of exemplary behaviour in military institutions, since their function is to systematize the general and common rules that structure them.

> Finally, there are establishments intended to serve as a refuge from the world, although they often also serve as places of instruction for the religious; examples of such institutions include abbeys, monasteries, convents and other cloisters. This classification of total institutions is not clear or exhaustive, nor is it of immediate analytical use, but it provides a purely denotative definition of the category as a concrete starting point (GOFFMAN, 2015, p.16).

Seeking to understand nursing homes as total institutions, we propose to describe the construction of a professional path that we followed through training in gerontology, developing different support practices through a university extension program for the elderly.

2.2. A journey through a university extension program for the elderly

Long-stay institutions for the elderly (ILPIs) are traditional nursing homes. This type of long-term care was established by Ministerial Order 2.854/2000[4] by the then Ministry of Social Development (MDS)[5] . This type of social assistance proposes comprehensive institutional care and must offer social, psychological, medical, physiotherapy and occupational therapy services.

Among some of the projects that I coordinate in the Universidade Aberta da Terceira Idade extension program at UERJ, we created a project called Asilar Atengao aos idosos. This project was designed so that the teams of residents in elderly health at UERJ, together with my team of scholarship students and social work interns, could look for philanthropic institutions in the nursing home care network that needed advice on making work plans feasible, monitoring the elderly in geriatrics and linking the nursing home to the resources of the elderly care network recommended by the public policies in force in Brazil.

One of the relevant prerogatives of the Asylum Care Project is to study the profiles of elderly people living in institutions, checking the reasons that led to their institutionalization, as well as studies on the assessment of functional and cognitive capacity, mobility and nutritional status. This project aims to develop an interdisciplinary action plan to support the issues intrinsic to the institutionalization of the elderly, to develop methodologies for specific approaches and to train professionals, technicians and managers of ILPIs.

The project was set up at UnATI/UERJ in 2006. Based on the catalog of nursing homes created by UnATI in 2002, we searched among the institutions already registered in the catalog for those that met the profile required by the project. The eligibility criteria for institutions to receive consultancy from UnATI were:

- Be philanthropic;
- Be up to date with all documentation;
- Have bylaws;
- Have an Advisory Board;

Amended by Ordinance 2.874/2000.

5 Ministry of Social Development (MDS) Program for the care of the elderly.

Be registered with the Municipal Social Assistance Council;
Be registered with the Municipal Council for the Elderly.

Once the institution had been chosen, we contacted the ILPI's social worker to find out whether she was interested in setting up a partnership with the State University of Rio de Janeiro.

We held a meeting to present the proposals drawn up by UnATI's team of technicians with a view to offering our expertise in the field of ageing. Once the parties had agreed, we started visiting the institution to collect data on the institutionalized elderly. We spoke to all the technical staff to find out about the possible difficulties encountered by the teams at these institutions with regard to the implementation of Ordinance 2874/2000, RDC 283/2005 and Law 10.741/2003, which lay down numerous care parameters to be respected in institutional spaces.

In 2007, as a member of the Rio de Janeiro State Council for the Defense of the Rights of the Elderly, I approached the Rio de Janeiro Public Prosecutor's Office with the intention of offering a technical cooperation agreement between UnATI/UERJ and the Public Prosecutor's Office, in order to promote, as part of the Asylum Care project, training for the professionals and managers of Long Stay Institutions for the Elderly (ILPI). The project was very well received by the supervisory institution and we started work that same year. Initially, we provided training for 220 professionals. That same year, we began to discuss the public policies recommended in Brazil and violence against the elderly. We got a favorable response from the evaluations we gave to the participants, who stressed the importance of the training space.

In the following years, we expanded our capacity until we reached the tenth year of training, in partnership with the MP-RJ, which took place in 2017, with a record attendance of 557 participants. This Training Seminar for ILPI Professionals and Managers is now part of UERJ's academic calendar and also of the actions carried out by the Public Prosecutor's Office with regard to policies for the care of the elderly.

In response to the good performance of the Asylum Care project and the questions it raised, I considered it relevant to present the proposal - to study the process of care offered in the institutionalization of aging and frail subjects, in a social, historical and psychoanalytic reflection - to the Professional Master's Degree in

Psychoanalysis, Health and Society, with a view to contributing to the improvement of social assistance and human rights actions in the field of institutionalization of the elderly. With this work, we intend to propose as a dissertation product a Training Manual for ILPI Managers and Professionals - The interface of gerontology with Care Practices, in order to deepen new horizons for work focused on caring for frail elderly people with degenerative diseases, with the aim of guaranteeing quality of life, dignity, rights and desires for the elderly who need to be supported by so-called comprehensive care institutions.

2.3. The reach of public policies and the practices of nursing homes

The care practices carried out in nursing homes merit a more in-depth discussion of the profile of people who are institutionalized. The nursing home, now known as the Long-Term Care Facility for the Elderly under the Social Assistance policy, is defined as a social facility providing comprehensive care that must ensure the health, dignity, social participation and protection of all elderly people who need it.

According to Monnerat and Souza (2011), the Organic Law on Social Assistance was published in 1993 and is defined as a Social Security policy, making up the Social Security tripe, along with Health and Social Security, linking the other policies in the social field. Social Assistance, unlike social security, is a non-contributory policy, meaning that it must serve all citizens who need it. It is carried out through integrated actions between public, private and civil society initiatives, with the aim of guaranteeing social protection for the family, childhood, adolescence and old age; support for needy children and adolescents; promoting integration into the labor market and rehabilitation and promoting integration into the community for people with disabilities and the payment of benefits to the elderly and people with disabilities (BRASIL, 2011).

According to Lima (2005), the Brazilian Society of Geriatrics and Gerontology (SBGG) adopted the term "Long-Stay Institution for the Elderly" (ILPI) to designate the type of institution formerly known as an Asylum. The SBGG defines it as an establishment for comprehensive institutional care, whose target public is people aged 60 or over, dependent or independent, who are unable to remain with their families or in a single-cell home. Based on the more contemporary concept of institutions for the elderly, Ordinance No. 73 of 2001 of the Ministry of Social Welfare and Social Security came into being, detailing all the components of an ILPI, as well as its procedures and care plans.

The National Policy for the Elderly (BRASIL, 1994) defines a nursing home as a residential facility for elderly people who have no family ties or are unable to provide for themselves, in order to meet their needs for housing, food, health and social interaction. It also states that such care should only take place in the event of the absence of a family group, abandonment, lack of financial resources of their own or of the family itself, without considering any other conditions, either on a temporary or permanent basis.

The Resolution of the Collegiate Board - RDC/ANVISA No. 283 of September 26, 2005, in its Article 1, approves the Technical Regulation that defines operating standards for Long Stay Institutions for the Elderly, of a residential nature, defines ILPI as "governmental and non-governmental institutions, of a residential nature, intended for the collective domicile of people aged 60 or over, with or without family support, in conditions of freedom, dignity and citizenship". (BRASIL, 2005).

The aim of RDC/ANVISA No. 283/2005[6] , was to establish the minimum operating standards for Long-Stay Institutions for the Elderly. The primary conditions it defines are listed in five definitions. They are:

Elderly caregiver - a person trained to help elderly people who have limitations in carrying out activities of daily living[7] ;

Elderly dependency - the condition of an individual who requires the assistance of people or special equipment to carry out activities of daily living;

Self-help equipment - any equipment or adaptation used to compensate for or enhance functional abilities, such as: canes, walkers, glasses, hearing aids and

---

6 Below is a summary of the main points of RDC/ANVISA no. 283/2005.

7 Elderly caregiver (CBO 5162-10) is currently an occupation according to the table of the Brazilian Code of Occupations of the Ministry of Labor. Congress is currently considering Bill 11 of 2016 to regulate the profession, which "creates and regulates the professions of Caregiver for the Elderly, Child Caregiver, Caregiver for People with Disabilities and Caregiver for People with Rare Diseases, and makes other provisions".

wheelchairs, among others with a similar function;

Degree of dependence of the elderly:

a) Dependency Level I - Independent elderly people, even if they require the use of self-help equipment;

b) Degree of Dependence II - Elderly people with dependence in up to three activities of self-care for daily living, such as: eating, mobility, hygiene, without cognitive impairment;

c) Dependency Level III - Elderly people with dependency who require assistance with all activities of self-care for daily living and/or cognitive impairment.

Autonomous individual - someone who has decision-making power and control over their life.

Long-stay institutions for the elderly are responsible for caring for the elderly, as defined in the technical regulations. The institution must provide for the exercise of the human rights (civil, political, economic, social, cultural and individual) of its residents. The institution must meet the following requirements, among others:

- Preserving the identity and privacy of the elderly, ensuring an environment of respect and dignity;
- Promote a welcoming environment;
- Promoting mixed living among residents with varying degrees of dependency;
- Promote the integration of the elderly in activities developed by the local community;
- Encourage the development of joint activities with people of other generations;
- Encourage and promote family and community participation in the care of elderly residents;
- Developing activities that encourage the autonomy of the elderly;
- Promoting leisure activities for the elderly, such as physical, recreational and cultural activities.

- Develop activities and routines to prevent and curb any kind of violence against people living there.

In addition to the legal requirements of documentation and registration with health control and rights defense entities, ILPIs must have a technical manager with a university degree and a postgraduate degree in Gerontology and Geriatrics.

For the care of residents, the law stipulates that for dependency level I, the institution must have one caregiver for every 20 elderly people on its staff, working 8 hours a day.

For dependency level II, one caregiver for every 10 elderly people per shift.

For dependency level III, one caregiver for every six elderly people per shift.

The physical space must meet ABNT standards in terms of access ramps, railings, flooring, lighting and other resources necessary for the well-being and safety of the institutionalized elderly and all the staff involved in the work provided at the ILPI.

In terms of health, the ILPI must draw up a comprehensive health care plan for the residents, in conjunction with the local health manager. The comprehensive health plan must be compatible with the principles of universalization, equity and comprehensiveness. The ILPI must indicate the health resources available to each resident at all levels of care, whether public or private. The ILPI must provide comprehensive care for the health of the elderly, addressing aspects of promotion, protection and prevention. It needs to contain information on the pathologies that occur and are prevalent among the elderly residents. When requested, the institution must provide proof of residents' mandatory vaccinations, as stipulated in the Ministry of Health's National Immunization Plan.

The Technical Manager is responsible for the medicines in use by the elderly, in compliance with the regulations of the Health Surveillance Authority regarding their safekeeping and administration. The institution must have written routines and procedures for caring for institutionalized elderly people.

The institution must immediately notify the local health authority of the following sentinel events: fall with injury and attempted suicide.

We have dealt extensively in this research with the existence of public policies and the care control procedures that an ILPI should have for institutionalized elderly people. However, we really need to contextualize the aging process from the point of view of subjective and social issues and the rites of passage through which individuals face their existence in contemporary society, leading up to their confinement in an institution.

2.4. Old age as a social category and its meanings

According to Borges (2007), the first known text on ageing dates back to 2,500 BC and was written by an Egyptian philosopher. The text laments the physical decrepitude that comes with advancing age. Beauvoir (1970/1990) points out that, although different societies have attributed different meanings to old age over the centuries, the theme of organic decline is recurrent and appears in the most varied communities in the history of human beings. According to Beauvoir (1970/1990), in the biblical accounts that reveal the beginnings of the Jewish people, from the 9th century onwards, old age is portrayed as a blessing and elderly men as people to whom respect is due. In Palestine, the oldest man ruled the family as long as his health was good.

Philipe Aries (1981, apud. DEBERT, 1998), in his book "Social History of the Child and the Family", provides one of the classic and most widespread examples of the study of the social construction of age categories. The historian demonstrates that in the Middle Ages children did not exist as a category, but were created in the thirteenth century, which resulted in the separation of children from adults. Children took part in the world of work and adult social life as soon as their physical abilities allowed, but over the years, the notion of childhood gradually developed and this group began to be treated as a specific problem. It was at this time that games, clothes and appropriate manners emerged to distinguish children from adults, and specific institutions were set up, such as schools, to prepare children for adulthood (FELIPE; SOUZA, 2014).

Reflecting on old age, we understand that studying only the biological processes of the human body, which result in aging, does not address the complexity of the process, as there are other factors that make up aging and that become essential in the search for answers about the phenomenon of old age. The philosopher Simone de Beauvoir (1990), in her work "Old Age", states that the subject cannot be understood without its totality, because it is not only a biological fact, but also a cultural fact.

At the age of 80, Plato returns to the issue at length in "The Laws". He often insists on the obligations of children towards their old parents, to whom they must speak respectfully, placing their wealth and their own person at their service. The dead ancestors are worshipped; the future ancestor is already sacred: "We can possess no object of worship more worthy of respect than a father or a grandfather, a mother or a grandmother oppressed by old age". (BEAUVOIR, 1970/1990, p. 136, apud BORGES, 2007).

From ancient Egypt to the Renaissance, the subject of old age was almost always treated in a stereotyped way; there were the same comparisons, the same adjectives. Old age is the winter of life. The whiteness of the hair and beard evokes snow, ice: there's a coldness to white which is offset by red - fire, ardor - and green, the color of plants, spring and youth. The clichés are perpetuated partly because the old suffer an immutable biological fate. But also, not being an agent of history, the old are of no interest - we don't take the trouble to study them in their truth. (BEAUVOIR, 1970/1990, p. 200).

Continuing with the historical processes and their contours with ageing, it is necessary to discuss the Industrial Revolution and the social manifestations that arose from it, characterized by the rural exodus. Workers who could no longer survive in the countryside migrated to the cities in search of work, making up the proletariat. Workers' work was hard and extremely exhausting, and much more oppressive for older workers. The literature of the time denounced, to a certain extent, the situation of the elderly who lived in poverty and the mistreatment they suffered, especially in texts that portrayed the situation of abandonment of the elderly in their own family, such as the novel *"La Terre"* by Zola, which tells the story of an old father who decides to divide his possessions among his children, because he can no longer work, and is plundered and murdered by them (BEAUVOIR, 1970/1990).

"Old age" as a social problem arose first and foremost in the working class because of

> the rapid extension, especially from the mid-19th century onwards, of the capitalist organization of work and the associated system of attitudes. Wages are assumed to remunerate only the strength invested in the work [...] the "old age" of the workers is then assimilated by the capitalist bosses to "invalidity", i.e. the "inability" to produce. [...] It was on the basis of this logic that the pension funds were set up by businessmen in order to reduce production costs, disposing in honorable conditions of elderly workers who earned too much for the income provided. (LENOIR, 1996, p.79).

According to Beauvoir (1970/1990), the bourgeoisie grew stronger and supplanted the aristocracy from an economic point of view, becoming more influential and powerful than the latter. The most influential representatives of the productive class were also the oldest, those who had accumulated experience and wealth over the years, thus establishing a "gerontocracy".

> DEBERT (1998) states that with regard to the chronology of life [...] the process of individualization, characteristic of modernity, had one of its fundamental dimensions in the institutionalization of the life course. One form of life, in which chronological age was practically irrelevant, was supplanted by another, in which age is a fundamental dimension of social organization. Stages of life are clearly defined and separated, and the boundaries between them are more strictly organized by chronological age. This growing institutionalization of the life course has involved practically every dimension of the family and work world, and is present in the organization of the production system, educational institutions, the consumer market and public policies that increasingly target specific age groups.

In the 19th century, new theories emerged about the causes of aging, some of which were still quite reductionist, such as the one that attributed aging to the involution of the sexual glands, or the one that determined, at the beginning of the 20th century, that human beings are as old as their arteries (BEAUVOIR, 1970/1990).

It was also at the beginning of the 20th century that geriatrics established itself as a specific field of medicine, consolidated by the physician Nascher, who in 1912 created the New York Geriatrics Society. From then on, research into senescence developed, meeting a numerically consistent demand, a consequence of the concentration of elderly people in large cities due to the growing industrialization process. But it wasn't until the 1930s that research into ageing took on a broader, less reductionist character and research associations on the subject multiplied in the United States (BEAUVOIR, 1970/1990).

Old age in contemporary times brings a new context to theories on aging. Beauvoir (1970/1990) demonstrated in her work that different societies characterize individuals in groups of old people according to a particular social organization. The roles related to social representations of old age are differentiated according to social status, the position the individual occupies in society and their purchasing power.

As we can see, exclusionary old age, produced by a capitalism of opportunities, does not gain visibility in this scenario. These old people, who are excluded from the capitalist system, need to make use of welfare benefits and the opportunities created by the advancement of certain social rights won since the 1988 Federal Constitution.

According to Borges (2007, apud HADDAD, 1986), aging in Brazil, given that it is a country that adopts a capitalist production structure, is a particularly complex phenomenon that cannot be analyzed solely from the perspective of individual aging.

Debert (2003) discusses the reprivatization of old age, which is the notion that being old or not is a choice that the individual makes. The author points out that in this model "being old is the result of a kind of moral lassitude, a problem of careless individuals who have been unable to engage in motivating activities and adopt the consumption of goods and services capable of combating ageing" (DEBERT, 203, p. 155). Such a conception completely ignores the real conditions of individuals in a class society and places the responsibility on the subject to remain connected to today's world, active, dynamic, "young in spirit".

Ageing today is seen as a process yet to be slowed down by capitalist ideology and even by international health and human rights policy bodies. *Anti-ageing"* medicine is present in pharmaceutical laboratories, clinics and the media, providing exceptional discoveries to slow down the ageing process.

Faced with all this rethinking of the aging process, it's worth diving into the paths proposed by Psychoanalysis.

2.5. The subject and desire in Freud's time of loss

Thinking about the elderly based on psychoanalytic theories makes me face a great challenge. In my studies of psychoanalysis, I noticed in Freud's writings that psychoanalysis would not be recommended for the elderly, as Freud (1898/1976) considered aging when people lived to be around 50 years old. Freud said that the time required for psychoanalytic treatment did not justify the investment.

When the work of analysis opens up new paths, we observe that the impulse has difficulty entering them. We call this behavior "id resistance". With such patients, the mental processes are fixed, immutable and rigid. This happens in old people (FREUD, 1937/1975, p. 12).

According to Torezan (et al, 2011, apud GARCIA-ROZA, 2001), the notions of subject and subjectivity constitute the very essence of what is known as the psychoanalytic field, which is made up of two regions that cannot be absolutely separated: the psychic apparatus and the drive field. Let's consider that from this point on, the fundamental point of Freudian theory focuses on the notion of the cleavage of subjectivity, through the formulation of the unconscious, regulated by laws different from those ordered by consciousness.

Still in Torezan (et al, 2011), another observation about the way the unconscious works, also of particular importance, is presented by Garcia-Roza (2000) when he says that Freud places psychoanalysis, from the beginning to the end of its journey, in the register of language, delimiting what he called the Freudian parabola, namely the emergence of the subject from language.

Torezan et al (2011) comment that the first of the two regions, the psyche, formed by the preconscious/conscious and unconscious systems, is usually understood as subjectivity itself. However, there is no way of completely separating one region from the other and when we talk about the psychic apparatus, we immediately refer to the drive representatives that make up this apparatus in its articulation with the register of the symbolic and, therefore, language. Thus, the second region, the field of impulses, is also implicated in the constitution of the first, the psychic apparatus.

It is pertinent to remember that the emergence of psychoanalysis takes place in the midst of modernity, when the discourse of science replaces theological discourse, and the notion of subjectivity becomes dominated by reason, and therefore led by consciousness (TOREZAN, et al, 2011, p. 529).

Following Freud's theories and thinking, it is pertinent to point out that in Freud (1900/2007), desire is characterized by an impulse in search of the reproduction of an original satisfaction, but in a hallucinatory way; in other words, the Father of Psychoanalysis refers to an object originally linked to satisfaction and no longer found, a lost object which is then represented in the Symbolic order. Thus, desire can be realized without ever being satisfied - unlike what happens with need, and always in a partial way, insofar as the encounter with the object, taken by desire circumstantially, also produces a remission of the mythical object lost forever, reopening dissatisfaction and relinking desire in its tireless circularity. At the heart of desire, then, is lack, because it is what continues to be present in reference to the lost object and, decisively, gives desire the status of unconscious and, therefore, foreign to the self. To this Freudian idea of unconscious desire that tends towards fulfillment, Lacan (1964/1988 apud TOREZAN, et al, 2011) articulated the phenomenological philosophical proposition of desire based on recognition, in which human desire is desire for the desire of the other. Roughly speaking, for psychoanalysis, what man desires is to be recognized by the desire of the other, to be loved, to be desired by the other, with the notion of desire being linked to that of an endless emptiness, for which there is no object to fill.

Freud (1929/2007), concerned with aspects between the subject and culture, advocated difficulties relating to social organization in the article "The Malaise in Culture". In this text, he states that one of the functions of culture is to regulate people's relationships with each other, but that its establishment depends on the renunciation of drive satisfaction, especially the renunciation of aggression. Thus, dissatisfaction is placed as a precondition for culture and referred to as cultural frustration. The article states that the loss of happiness, through the feeling of guilt engendered by culture, is the price paid for cultural evolution.

Freud (1929/2007) considers life to be very heavy, and that suffering threatens us in three ways: the decay of the body itself, the outside world and relationships with others. In addition to highlighting the suffering that comes from human relationships, there is the observation that the purpose of avoiding suffering is greater than that of seeking pleasure, despite the fact that the search for unlimited satisfaction is a tempting rule of conduct. Freud chooses three forms

main ways of reducing this suffering: distractions that make our misery seem small, substitute satisfactions that reduce it, and narcotics that make us insensitive to it.

For Castilho (2011), old age perceived as an inexorable event in life implies sudden losses of significant references, sometimes concomitant, which cause "tearing" pain and are often presented in discourse as irreplaceable. For some elderly people, these events can be seen in their speech as a trauma or as the result of a fate, an obscure destiny that emphasizes pain and suffering.

> Old age, with its hardships, comes to everyone. I'm not rebelling against the universal order. After all, I've lived more than seventy years. I've had enough to eat. I've enjoyed many things - the company of my wife, my children, the sunset. I've watched the plants grow in spring. Every now and then I've had a helping hand to squeeze. Once in a while I met a human being who almost understood me. What more could I want? (FREUD, 1926/2011, s/p.)

Thus, according to MESSY (1993), all the losses experienced throughout a subject's existence indicate marks that structure their self: the loss of milk teeth in children and the move towards adolescence. The loss of virginity in young people is a milestone that brings them closer to adulthood. For adults, the menopause in women, retirement and the loss of close people of the same chronological age (MESSY, 1993 apud BALDIN, 2012).

With regard to finitude, Castilho (2011) says that common sense sees the link between old age and death as almost natural. Freud (1915), however, evaluates our attitude towards death as the fact that each of us is convinced, in our unconscious, of our own immortality, thus making the reference to death so present in the discourse of the elderly enigmatic. The fact is that conviction in one's own immortality wavers under certain circumstances. This is what happens in the face of a valuable, significant loss, experienced as a loss in the self (FREUD, 1915), but also in situations with the value of trauma that confront us with our own finitude, regardless of chronological age.

2.6. Cinema and psychoanalysis as analytical tools

While lying on the diva, Freud encouraged patients to relate their concerns, allowing free association. They initially described their issues through dreams. Today, films, film impressions and dreams are part of the analysis process. On the subject of free association in psychoanalysis, Froemming (2002) says that free association arose from the criticism of hypnosis and the cathartic method in the treatment of hysteria cases, since Anna O. (FREUD, 1893/1976). The method consists of indiscriminately expressing all the thoughts that occur to the mind, either from a given element (word, number, image from a dream) or spontaneously. It is widely used in dream interpretation (FREUD, 1900/1976).

According to Lemos (2014), at the end of the 19th century and the beginning of the 20th century, there was a scientific, social and cultural upsurge of major proportions. Allergic to the positivist promises, or in opposition to them, social events of great global repercussion were engendered, including the invention of the cinematograph by the *Lumiere* brothers and the proposition of psychoanalysis by Freud, among others.

Researching notes on cinema and its history, I identified the creation of cinema as associated with Plato's Myth of the Cave.

In Plato's Myth of the Cave, the philosopher sets out his vision of the human condition in relation to reality as a whole. A huge cave, connected to the outside world by a long passage that prevents any daylight from entering the cave. Looking at the back wall with your back to the cave entrance, you see a row of prisoners. Their limbs are chained, as are their necks, so that they can't move their heads and can't look at each other. Behind them in the cave, there is a large fire and because of the light, the prisoners can see shadows of statues being carried on the back wall (CANDIDO, 2011).

What would happen, asks Plato, if someone freed the prisoners? Although sore from years of immobility, a prisoner would start walking towards the entrance to the cave and, coming across the ascending path, enter it.

At first, he would be completely blind, because the fire is actually sunlight, and he would be completely dazzled by it. Then, getting used to the brightness, he would see the men carrying the statues and, continuing along the path, he would see the things themselves, discovering that, all his life, he had seen only shadows of images (the shadows of the statues projected onto the bottom of the cave) and that only now is he contemplating reality itself.

Freed and aware of the world, the prisoner would return to the cave, be bewildered by the darkness, tell the others what he had seen and try to free them. What would happen to him on his return? The other prisoners would mock him, and his experience would be incomprehensible to those people whose language would only have shadows and echoes as references: "All they can see is the wall in front of them". (CANDIDO, 2011).

The way to begin to see this allegory is to see ourselves, as imprisoned in our own bodies, with other prisoners like us as company, and all of us, as unable to discern real beings from each other, or at least our own real being. Our direct experience is not of reality itself, but of what is in our minds. The Platonist cave is sometimes compared to the darkroom, described as a door whose only opening is a tiny hole in one of its walls.

On the opposite wall is drawn an exact reproduction, but inverted, of what could be seen outside.

Plato's Cave has also been compared to a movie theater: the spectators being the prisoners in chains and the images on the screen, the shadows projected onto the walls of the cave (CANDIDO, 2011).

According to Lemos (2014), the articulation between psychoanalysis and cinema has been marked by polemics and controversies from the outset. According to Lacoste (1992), Freud traveled to the United States of America in 1909 to deliver his famous lectures at Clark University. On that occasion, the cinema was presented to him as a novelty that could be used in the alleged teaching and dissemination of psychoanalysis.

A little later, enjoying the acceptance and popularity achieved by psychoanalysis, in 1924, Freud received a visit from Samuel Goldwyn, founder of Paramount and creator of the Company. Then, Metro Goldwyn Mayer, proposing a partnership in a film with a romantic theme, in which he (Freud) would receive the initial sum of one hundred thousand American dollars for the dissemination and use of psychoanalytic concepts in cinema. Even though Samuel Goldwyn crossed the Atlantic Ocean just to make the proposal, it was turned down, and Freud remained resistant to the use of psychoanalysis associated with the seventh art (LACOSTE, 1992, apud LEMOS, 2014).

In his work, "Malaise in Civilization" (FREUD, 1930[1929]/1987), he speaks of the feelings of guilt and happiness as superfluous, even calling his reflections an old man's pastime. According to Aumont (et. al. 1994/2011), the primary identification in cinema is that by which the spectator identifies with his own gaze and feels himself to be the focus of the representation, as the privileged, central and transcendental subject of the vision. "It is he who sees this landscape from this unique point of view, it could also be said that the representation of this landscape is organized entirely for a precise and unique place which is precisely that of his eye". (AUMONT, et. al. 1994/2011, p. 260).

According to Aumont and Marie (2009 apud LEMOS, 2014), in the 1970s, under the aegis of the development of the social sciences, which opposed those who advocated a critical approach to texts of a traditional nature and those who accepted only the manifest text, psychoanalysis became the subject of heated debates. According to the authors, "these texts address the subjective effects of filmic language, which, with the support of semiotic-linguistic readings, propose a theory of the subject, aspects neglected in other approaches" (AUMONT; MARIE, 2009). It is also in this direction that I advocate an approximation between psychoanalysis and cinema.

To better understand the behavior of people imprisoned in closed institutions, I turned to Luis Bunuel's masterful film "The Exterminating Angel". In this movie, a couple from the elite of aristocratic society invite a group of friends to their luxurious mansion for dinner. But after the event, they discover that they are trapped in a room. There is nothing physical, like bars, to hold them, but at the same time, no one can get out or in: something is holding them hostage. As the days go by, all the masks and social conventions disappear, giving way to their most primitive instincts.

I intend to use the tools of cinema and psychoanalysis to investigate what exactly defines old age and the anxieties of growing old, together with the anguish of memory loss, confinement and the proximity of death, based on the aforementioned film.

What should determine old age be in the realm of advancing age, biological and social aspects and organic wear and tear? Perhaps an analysis of reminiscence could shed some light.

For Santos and Carlos (2011), longevity in contemporary times, as a phenomenon resulting from life changes and advances in science in relation to health care, leads us to reconsider the fact that ageing, like the unconscious, never ceases to register. Thus, the unconscious of old people continues to record their history, beyond chronological time, in a game of hide and seek, between past memories and present recollections, and through the failure to resolve or elaborate obscure points that insist on producing symptoms, as a result of guilt that is still active, due to the force of repression.

Still according to Lacan (1999, apud SANTOS; CARLOS, 2011), the unconscious leaves open the re-signification that can be re-inscribed by the signifying chain. We cannot neglect the idea that there is still an unconscious that arises from the formations of the unconscious, in other words, symptoms, dreams, failed acts, forgetfulness that mark the real of the body in its losses and functional changes with the passage of time or age (LACAN, 1999).

Next, we'll look at the cinematic universe by describing Luis Bunuel's "The Exterminating Angel". We will then look at the analogy between the film and the issues that make up the social construction of an old people's home.

2.7. The Exterminating Angel movie - scene one (analogy from the movie)

Luis Bunuel Portoles was born on February 22, 1900, in the village of Calanda, in the province of Teruel, Aragao, Spain. He was the son of Leonardo Bunuel Gonzales, a wealthy landowner who had made his fortune in Cuba with a hardware business, and Maria Portoles Cerezuela. Shortly afterwards, the family settled in Saragoqa and only went to Calaqa during Holy Week, the summer holidays. Luis was the eldest of seven brothers and sisters, with whom he had a happy, healthy and carefree childhood, in contact with the rich countryside of his land. From an early age, he had a great sensitivity to the extraordinary, and was easily enchanted by animals, plants and natural phenomena, which he observed attentively, imbued with a paid religiosity. It was also during his childhood that he acquired an enormous fascination with death, when he inadvertently came across a putrefying donkey in a ditch.

In 1908, he saw his first movie in a Zaragoza cinema. He studied at a Jesuit school, whose childhood would be felt for the rest of his life. In his teens he lost his faith, became anti-clerical and atheist, and in 1915 he was expelled from school, having finished his secondary studies at the Saragoqa Institute.

In 1917, Bunuel went to study in Madrid. He met a number of Spanish and international intellectuals in the fields of literature, arts and sciences and lived with many of those who were part of the famous Generation of '27, learning about the artistic and literary avant-gardes of the time - cubism, dadaism and surrealism. It was at this time that he became the companion of three bohemian friends who were of fundamental importance to him: Pepin Bello, Frederico Garcia Lorca and Salvador Dali.

In 1920, he founded the first Spanish film club. In 1924, after attending several university courses without much conviction, he ended up with a degree in History.

In 1925, he went to live in Paris, where he studied film and worked as an assistant director to several filmmakers.

In January 1929, Bunuel and Dali, using the surrealist method, wrote the guide for the film that would end up being titled *"Un chien andalou"* (An Andalusian Dog).

Bunuel's works contain all the basic themes of his entire oeuvre: mad love, anti-clericalism, rebellion and non-conformity in the face of the established and the conventional, a yearning for transcendence, expressed in dreamlike and hallucinatory images, full of harshness, corrosive black humor and intoxicating candor.

In 1930, he traveled to Hollywood, hired by Metro Goldwyn Mayer as an observer, with the aim of familiarizing himself with the American production system.

Bunuel returned to Spain after the proclamation of the republic and, financed by his anarchist friend Ramon Acin, directed a documentary in 1933, *"Las Hurdes, tierra sin pan",* which described in a raw way the daily life and ancestral customs of a deeply miserable Spanish village in an almost savage state. The images and facts described were so extraordinary and unreal that they ended up giving the film a truly surrealistic feel. It was a scandal, displeasing the Spanish government, which banned it, much to Bunuel's disappointment, for giving a corrupt image of Spain abroad.

During the Spanish Civil War, he went into exile in France, leaving in 1938 for the United States. In 1941, he worked as an advisor and head of editing for the Museum of Modern Art (MoMA) in New York.

In 1946, after having worked in Hollywood, he left for Mexico, where he made major contributions to world cinema.

After filming the masterpiece **The Exterminating Angel in** Mexico in 1962, he returned to France and began filming other great works in the country.

In 1970 he returned to Spain and in 1972 filmed **Discreet Charm of the Bourgeoisie,** which won the Oscar for Best Foreign Film.

In 1982, he published his excellent autobiography, *"Mon Dernier Soupir"* (**My Last Sigh**), in which, close to death, he reaffirmed his convictions and recounted his memories, despite his increasing problems with amnesia.

He died in Mexico City on July 29, 1983 and, according to his wishes, was cremated and his ashes scattered.

The Exterminating Angel - scene one (movie analogy)

When I chose Bunuel's work to contextualize my work on institutions for the care of the elderly, I realized that I could combine two great pleasures in a single theme. I love Bunuel's work because I see him as a transgressor of Marxist ideology, using fantastical surrealism to criticize capital and its idle bourgeoisie. Scenarios brought up in Bunuel's work, such as confinement, hypocrisy, farce, resistance and social subversion, are intrinsically linked to the universe of my research as well as to my theoretical framework.

As described above, the movie shows that mysteriously, after a lavish dinner party hosted by a very wealthy bourgeois couple, none of the guests manage to leave the mansion. Over the course of the next few days, all the masks created by social positions fall away and give way to the wildest instincts that can spring up in human beings when they are oppressed, enclosed or subjected to controversial and stigmatized disciplinary orders.

The Exterminating Angel - take - scene one.

The film begins its first shot with Christian images and the representation of religious dogmas that are probably present in the Christian Jewish culture built into the social formation of individuals.

In scene one of the movie **The Exterminating Angel,** I observe that the servants of the mansion, as in closed institutions, subvert the order of the owners of the house in a space between two very different groups: bourgeois, masters of the social order, and proletarians, rebellious and impulsive.

In scene one of the film, the unease in social relations begins to appear as soon as the group of bourgeoisie realize that they have no prospects at the dinner party. The emergence of silent chaos begins to take hold of that setting which, although luxurious, has an implicit sense of disorder. It's clear from the owners of the mansion that they want to impose order on their employees at all times, but there is evidence of social tensions dampened by the imposition of disciplinary rules.

When the confinement begins in the scene, there is an attempt to subvert the social order when the guests remain in the room for hours, giving up etiquette to spend the night in the same physical space, without any formality.

In his work, Goffman (2015) deals with the rigidity of institutional orders and compliance with rules, under penalty of punishment and social exclusion.

In scene one, there is resistance to imposed orders and the confinement that comes from environments where the persecutory imaginary is characterized by rules that are described in gestures represented by the characters idealized by Bunuel. We will continue to analyze the film in the following two chapters.

3. PERSPECTIVES ON INSTITUTIONALIZED OLD AGE

In this chapter, we analyze the notion of asylum and the institutionalization of old age, initially situating historical and social dimensions and reflecting on the regulatory framework of public policies for ILPI's and social rights in contemporary times. A theoretical, reflective and critical look at the subject will be taken through the concepts of total institution and the mortification of the self, in Goffman's view, and the notions of power, disciplinary power and biopolitics in Foucault, with an analysis of two film productions that will illustrate the study undertaken.

3.1. The historical and social construction of asylums in Brazil

In order to better contextualize long-stay institutions for the elderly, it is essential that we look at the historical aspects that have been fundamental elements in the construction of the social ageing process in our society, through customs and practices that have determined the scenario of institutions for the reception of individuals burdened by stigmas and the process of exclusion latent in Brazilian society, from the 19th century to the present day.

According to Filizzola (1972), the history of asylums began in 1790, when Count Resende arrived in Rio de Janeiro to become the 5th Viceroy. Viceroy. A man of avant-garde ideas for his time, the Viceroy decided to have built what the author considers to be the first institution for old people in the country: The House of the Invalids. This was located on Rua Nova Sao Lourengo, which today bears the name Rua dos Invalidos. It was a farmhouse whose land occupied an area equivalent to the block formed by Rua dos Invalidos, Senado, Relagao and do Amaral, in the city center. The author explains that the new institution was intended to collect "soldiers who had grown old in years and were tired of work", who had come from Portugal for the 1762 campaign and who "through their service were worthy of a restful old age" (FILIZZOLA, 1972, p.27 apud SANTOS, 2007).

According to Filizzola (1972), "the emergence of such a House was the result of the ideas of an extraordinary man" who decided to go against all the rules of the time and create an institution in Brazil (FILIZZOLA, 1972, p. 44). The Count of Resende would have been moved by French ideals, inspired by the work of Louis XIV, who had erected the Hotel *des Invalides* in Paris for the heroes of the French campaigns. Having started operating in 1794, the Casa dos Invalidos was to be short-lived. With the arrival of the court in 1808, King João decided to give the house to his private doctor, the Baron of Alvaiazar, and the invalids were transferred to the Santa Casa de Misericordia. Exactly who and how many these "invalids" were, as well as more details about how the institution functioned, is information that the author is unable to obtain, as apparently there are very few sources relating to the short period of operation of the institution.

For Santos (2007), the 19th century was marked by three moments that allow us to construct a small panorama of the social values involved in the treatment of urban poverty: its first decades, when charity is the main guiding force behind actions on poverty; the second half of the century, when philanthropy and social medicine inspire the state in practices of repression and institutionalization; and, finally, the end of the century and the beginning of the 20th century, when the criteria for differentiating and institutionalizing the "dangerous classes" are better delineated. At this time, destitute old age emerges as a category that classifies and separates certain individuals from the agglomeration of types that make up urban beggary, assigning them a privileged place of assistance: the old people's home.

Santos (2007) writes that in Rio de Janeiro, in August 1854, the Asilo de Mendicidade, known as the Albergaria, was founded. Its purpose was to receive and provide shelter for all the beggars found in the streets, churchyards, plagues, etc. It was located in Rua de Santa Luzia and had a capacity for 70 beggars, with a room for men with 40 seats and 30 for women. Beggars were thus given a special institution whose purpose was to collect and sort the indigent population, separating the sick and disabled from criminals. Less than a year after its inauguration, the institution began to deal permanently with begging. The justification was the threat to public health.

In order to better contextualize the end of the 19th century, in terms of the social transformations experienced by Brazilian society, Santos (2007) records in his research that the 19th century brought several transformations to the way of life and the organization of society. Santos (2007) reports that some authors particularly highlight transformations in family composition as decisive for a change in values in relation to old age. According to Gilberto Freyre (1990), the social changes that accompanied the transition from the patriarchal society of colonial Brazil to the new urban order of the 19th century stripped old people of the prestige they had enjoyed. The extended family became nuclear, and the figure of the elderly patriarch, the highest authority in the colonial family, lost his mythical power.

With regard to the changes that came with the 20th century, Santos (2007) points out that institutional practices were not restricted to miserable old people. In 1909, the Asilo Sao Luiz created a pavilion for old people who were not destitute, but who wished to be housed on a monthly basis. It seems that at that time, the institutionalization of old age was no longer just charity, but also a source of income. At that moment, it was not helplessness that was being assisted, but old age itself.

Old age began the 20th century closely linked to nursing homes. In this century, nursing homes were philanthropic in nature. Most of them were religiously oriented, where elements such as 'charity' and 'assistance' took over. During this period, asylums did not get closer to society and there was an apparent perception that society should not know what happened in these places. In 1996, a scandal broke out in Rio de Janeiro involving a shelter for the elderly. This event generated a new paradigm in nursing home care after the death of a significant number of elderly people who were cared for by the institution. For a more precise account of the facts, I quote Groismam (1999b):

> May 30, 1996 can be considered a milestone for understanding the "problem" of the institutionalization of old age in Brazil at the end of this century. That morning, Rio de Janeiro woke up to the following headline in its largest newspaper: "bacteria kills ten elderly people in clinic". The case of the Clinica Santa Genoveva had come to light and would occupy the main pages of the media for almost two months (GROISMAM, 1999b, p. 165).

After this article, new facts emerged. What had happened at the Santa Genoveva Clinic, following complaints from some of the staff, were episodes of mistreatment. The headline appeared in the newspapers and it is known that 84 elderly people died in this tragic episode.

For Groisman (1999b), the world of institutional practices regarding old age would appear with all its contradictions. With its 340 beds and countless deaths, Santa Genoveva became a point of tension for the meanings of old age in Brazil, momentarily illuminating some facets of the power play present in the complex issue of the institutionalization of old age.

Faced with the revelation of an absurd situation involving frail, sick and helpless old people, the Public Prosecutor's Office opens an investigation to uncover what nursing homes were and how they functioned in that historical period of this narrative.

Groisman (1999b) argues in his article that in order to do this, however, we would have to broaden our analytical spectrum and place the institutionalization of old age in a historical perspective. It would be necessary to go back in time and think about the genesis of this type of institution. Look for a time when the founding of old people's homes was a source of pride for society and the newspapers celebrated it. The author refers to the creation of the Sao Luiz Asylum for Destitute Old People, founded in Rio de Janeiro on September 4, 1890.

We will revisit the São Luiz Asylum for destitute old people in the analysis of the documentary "Come Sweet Death", which will be analyzed in this theoretical research.

3.2.Regulatory framework and public policies for ILPIs and social rights today

According to Veras (1994), the longevity of the population is a worldwide phenomenon that has major social and economic repercussions. However, this process differs from country to country. Developing countries like Brazil are characterized by the speed with which the absolute and relative increase in the adult and elderly populations has been changing the population pyramid.

According to Veras (1994), the processes of demographic and epidemiological transition in Brazil are clearly heterogeneous and are largely associated with the unequal social conditions observed in the country. The elderly population is a very different group from each other and from other age groups, both from the point of view of social conditions and demographic and epidemiological aspects.

With this in mind, it is extremely important to contextualize the social rights guaranteed to individuals who have crossed the 60-year mark since the promulgation of the Federal Constitution in 1988, which guaranteed a legal provision for this age group of the Brazilian population.

According to Carvalho (2011), the National Policy for the Elderly (PNI) establishes social rights, guarantees of autonomy, integration and participation of the elderly over 60 in society, as a legal instrument of citizenship itself. In order to achieve these aims, essential guidelines were defined: home care; stimulating medical training in the field of gerontology; political-administrative decentralization; and the dissemination of studies and research on aspects related to the elderly and ageing. Its principles state that: family, society and the state have a duty to ensure that the elderly have all the rights of citizenship, guaranteeing their participation in the community, defending their dignity, well-being and right to life; the ageing process concerns society in general and should be the subject of knowledge and information for all; the elderly must not be discriminated against in any way; and in the application of the law, the economic, social and regional differences and, in particular, the contradictions between rural and urban areas in Brazil must be taken into account by the public authorities and society in general.

Looking at the text of the National Policy for the Elderly, its guidelines state that public bodies should encourage home care for the elderly and that priority should be given to care for the elderly by their families, to the detriment of nursing homes, except for those elderly people who do not have or need the conditions to maintain their own survival.

For our research, it is interesting to note that the National Policy for the Elderly (PNI), encourages the creation of alternative forms of care for the elderly, such as Casalar, Republica de idosos, Centro de convivencia, Centro dia, Atendimento domiciliar. Such facilities should fulfill an extremely important function in view of the prospects for population growth in Brazil. It is worth noting that the text of the law does not indicate funding for these modalities, nor does it encourage their implementation in the organization of public policies in the area of social rights for elderly individuals who need them.

According to Ordinance 2.874/2000 of the then Ministry of Social Development, the modalities of care for vulnerable groups, including the elderly, are defined in its text. Below we will discuss the definition of the modalities according to the Ordinance.

Characterization of the service:

Comprehensive institutional care - this is care provided in institutions known as: shelters, nursing homes, homes and rest homes, during the day and night, for elderly people in situations of abandonment, without families or unable to live with their families. These institutions must guarantee the provision of care services, hygiene, food and shelter, health, physiotherapy, psychological support, occupational activities, leisure, culture and others, according to the needs of the users. The institution is also responsible for making constant efforts to rebuild family ties that will enable the elderly person to return to their family.

Residence with a foster family - this is care provided by families registered and trained to offer shelter to elderly people in situations of abandonment, without a family or unable to live with their families. This service will be continuously supervised by the managing bodies.

Casalar Residence - is an alternative residence for small groups of up to eight elderly people, with suitable furniture and a qualified person to support the elderly person's daily needs. It is mainly aimed at elderly people with some kind of dependency.

Residence in Republics - Elderly republics are an important alternative form of residence for independent elderly people, also organized in small groups, depending on the number of users, and co-funded with resources from pensions, long-term care benefits, monthly income for life and others. In some cases, the Republica can be run on a self-management basis.

Day care - is a care strategy in specialized institutions, where the elderly person stays for eight hours a day, receiving health care, physiotherapy, psychological support, occupational activities, leisure and other services, according to the needs of the users. It is important because the elderly can be cared for during the day and return home at night and because it allows them to maintain their family ties. The capacity of the day center is variable and must always be appropriate to the quality of the service, in accordance with specific standards.

Home care - is care provided to elderly people with some level of dependency, by caregivers, in at least two visits a week to the elderly person's own home. It is designed to support the elderly and their families in their day-to-day activities, with a view to promoting, maintaining and/or recovering autonomy, remaining in their own homes, strengthening family and neighborhood ties and improving their quality of life.

Care in a Social Center - consists of activities carried out in a specific physical space, equipped with infrastructure that allows the elderly and their families to attend for at least 16 hours a week, preferably with a daytime stay of eight hours a day, to enjoy a program that aims to promote sociability, the development of skills, information, updating, educational, artistic, sports and leisure activities, among others. The community center must offer a series of planned and organized activities to be enjoyed by the elderly and their families, with a participatory management model through a management council, which will establish the program.

Social group care / Conviver Project - consists of activities carried out with independent elderly people in physical spaces available in the community, such as churches, schools, community centers, health centers, multipurpose centers and others, through regular attendance of at least 6 hours a week and adapted to the possibilities of the groups, with a program drawn up based on the interests of the elderly. As it is a community facility, the activities developed are organized according to the possibilities of the infrastructure, focusing on social services. The coexistence groups are methodological strategies whose objectives are: group nucleation, activities including sightseeing tours, inter-group meetings, recreational, labor and artistic activities, with the aim of expanding social relations, as well as enabling the autonomy of the groups, in spaces close to where the elderly live.

In order to guarantee fundamental rights, Law 10.741/2003, the Statute of the Elderly, was instituted. It regulates the rights of all people aged 60 or over and should guarantee dignity, in addition to the social rights already advocated in Law 8.842/1994 (PNI), from the perspective of living in a community, increasing physical health and mental health.

Considering Article 52 of the Statute of the Elderly, we can then analyze the object of our research, reviewing the socio-historical aspects of the institutionalization of the elderly. In this article, the Statute of the Elderly assigns the Public Prosecutor's Office, Health Surveillance and councils (municipal, state and national) the task of inspecting establishments that cater for the elderly, imposing administrative penalties on those who fail to comply with the legal determinations, according to the nature and seriousness of the infraction committed. I believe that it is not only in the legal system that we need to consider changes to the spaces where the elderly are sheltered, but that we need to intensify social actions that allow the various social spaces through which people relate to each other to intersect. Shelters for the elderly should not be enough in themselves, but should establish a permanent dialog with the subjects' daily lives. In order to broaden this reflection, however, we need to delve into Erving Goffmam's (2015) thoughts on total institutions so that we can seek an analytical reflection with a good critical bias in order to build a new paradigm for institutions for the elderly in Brazil.

3.3.Goffman's characteristics of total institutions

Goffman (2015) defines the total institution "as a place of residence and work where a large number of similarly situated individuals, separated from the wider society for a considerable period of time, lead a closed and formally administered life". (GOFFMAN, 2015, p. 11).

When Goffman (2015) defines the asylum as a total institution, we feel the need to reveal this space of confinement, taking into account the frail, old bodies forgotten by society. The observations on institutions for the elderly recorded below are consolidated reports drawn from observations made in professional practice.

First of all, I'm going to use Goffman (2015, p. 23) to describe "the world of the inmate in the total institution". In my professional practice with institutions for the elderly, I realize that when they arrive at the institution, they bring with them a diffuse perception of what the institution is like and what the customs there are. They bring with them cultural, social and religious habits and the individuality characteristic of the formation of their personalities and desires built up over the course of their lives. The total institutions for the elderly do not seem to promote the complete and immediate cultural replacement of the habits brought by the elderly, but with the permanence of the elderly possibly until death, all cultural habits may be replaced by new habits and by reminiscences brought up as good memories built up by a course of life that can sustain the anguish and certainty of finitude. "The newcomer arrives at the establishment with a conception of himself made possible by certain stable social arrangements in his domestic world," says Goffman (2015, p.24).

Closed institutions such as asylums, for example, are surrounded by walls that already portray a climate of confinement, where the doors are only opened with the express authorization of the head of the institution or an individual appointed for this purpose. The old people who live there carry out certain rituals delegated to them without any question as to why they are doing the task delegated to them by the head of nursing or by caregivers who carry out routine tasks. In many cases, there is no bond or feeling in the tasks, just a mechanical "doing".

The inmates are treated in the same way, as if they were coming out of the same structure to receive the same daily tasks prescribed by a big boss. The activities planned by the administration are compulsory and are set down in a single bureaucratic plan established by the institution, created to meet official assumptions and the families responsible for the elderly in the institution. The control of the human needs of the inmates is implemented every day without resizing the variables required by the individual dynamics of each subject. There is also control and vigilance among the inmates over the occasional disoriented person who wants to break the established rules by running away or failing to fulfill their daily tasks. The latter is under the strict gaze of caregivers with a more authoritarian profile and harsher language, so that the inmate feels fearful or afraid of breaking the established rules.

Like Goffman's (2015) description of total institutions, the group of inmates live their lives in the asylum with almost no contact with the outside world. The institution tends to label the inmates, often seeing them as bitter, grouchy, hostile, authoritarian and aggressive people, without contextualizing that individual's universe and what led them to arrive at that institution to end their days.

In these closed institutions, the roles of social control are well defined. There is the big boss, then there is the nursing team, the team of technicians who just carry out their activities of caring for and maintaining the health of the inmates and the team of subordinates such as kitchen staff, laundry, janitorial and cleaning staff. All of them seem not to question the confinement of people and accept that the confinement and imprisonment imposed there may seem "normal". Each of these groups tends to know the other through limited and hostile stereotypes. Old people seem to see the leaders as the ultimate authority, sometimes arbitrary, but condescending to human old age.

In this contradiction of social roles[8] , the old people inside tend to feel inferior, weak, sad and accommodated to the *"status quo"* imposed by the institution and the managers correct and compliant with the established rules, aimed at protecting and caring for the institutionalized old people.

In his analysis of the phenomenon of total institutions, Goffman (2015) defines that the concept of power exercised by these institutions is eminently modelling, rigid, repressive and mutilating of the self, in order to re-establish a resocializing mission.

In total institutions such as those for the elderly, there is a distancing between the elderly and the individuals linked to the power hierarchies of the institution, as well as the individuals who carry out the orders and services, as if they would never be in the place of the elderly institutionalized there. This is how different cultural and social worlds develop in the same living space.

Another analysis considered relevant in Goffman (2015) deals with the mortification of the self, where the first refers to institutions that impose as a rule that individuals lose their autonomy when they are interned in these spaces, such as always being accompanied by someone from the team who must perform the task of being close to the individuals at times or tasks inherent in the institutional routine. The other conduct is to provoke in inpatients the sensation of feeling demeaned by the system imposed by the institution and self-mortification, i.e. being weakened by the feeling of renouncing actions and wills. These processes aim to control the daily lives of a significant number of individuals in a restricted space.

In nursing homes, the planning and execution of leisure, social and family activities is not continuous and can flow as a result of a demand made by inspection bodies to protect the legislation governing institutions for the elderly or a complaint

---

8 "By social roles we can roughly define the representations of characters that we create and recreate according to the social relationships we maintain in our daily lives, the setting, our previous experiences and our future expectations, what Schutz (1989) called the "meaningful context" (Sinnzusammenhang) (...) According to Goffman we represent social roles consciously and also unconsciously. For him, "the traditions of a personal role will lead you to give a deliberate impression of a certain species, and yet it is possible that you have neither consciously nor unconsciously intended to create such an impression" (GOFFMAN, 1999, p. 15 apud BODART; MADALENA, 2012, p. 10).

from a family member concerned about the feeling of apathy and melancholy of their institutionalized elderly person.

In order to circumvent the rigid rules imposed on the confinement of old people, the subordinates receive "gifts" or treats in monetary value to bring comfort and joy to the old people who are trying to resist confinement as a way of removing the suffering and anguish they feel from living in a closed institution. It's worth noting that the rules are circumvented in collusion with other elements linked to the institution, but who will use the trust established between old people and subordinates to subvert the rules in exchange for compensatory treats.

For Goffman (2015), the process of mortification is accompanied by the "system of privileges". This system translates into a set of internalized auguries in institutional conduct and customs. The first relates to prohibitions related to the conduct of the inmate; the second relates to a number of clearly defined privileges that are obtained in exchange for obedience to the leaders; the third item is related to the procedures linked to the punishments that must be applied as a result of disobedience to the rules imposed by the institution.

The family is another interesting element when analyzing the context of a total institution. It is the vehicle for the internment of elderly individuals, alleging cognitive decline, social isolation, domestic disorder due to functional fragility or other emotional and social reflexes that are still veiled in family relationships.

When the process of institutionalization begins, family members show themselves to be solicitous and concerned about the adaptation of the elderly, but soon afterwards the routine of confinement gives way to family discomfort caused by guilt over the act of institutionalization, and visits from children and grandchildren begin to spiral out of control until, in many cases, their presence in the institution disappears completely.

Let's go back to the processes of mortification of the self. These are defined by Goffman (2015, pp.24-39) as "the processes by which a person's 'self' is mortified and are relatively standardized in total institutions". Here I emphasize the importance of demonstrating them. When contextualizing an institution for the elderly as a total institution, one of the aspects of confinement that make up the universe of these institutions are the architectural barriers, because when the elderly individual enters this space divided between the real world and the totalitarian world constructed from institutional norms, rules and procedures, the individual is no longer recognized as a subject of desires and attitudes, but becomes an individual without expression in the face of the impositions prescribed by the processes of institutional care and protection. I can see that there is a predominance of the process described by Goffman (2015), when the old person is brought to the institution without having been consulted. Another element that makes us understand asylums as total institutions is the bureaucratic and rigid procedures by which institutions manage their rules and ways of acting in order to maintain order and procedures unchanged for years.

Goffman (2015) also deals with "adaptation tactics" in his analysis. In this context, the author works with a number of categories: the tactic of withdrawal, in which the internee stops paying attention to everything, with the exception of events related to their body. The other tactic is the so-called "intransigence tactic", in which the inmate intentionally defies the institution by refusing to follow the rules imposed there. Another tactic described by the author concerns the "adaptation tactic", which is used as a reference point to demonstrate how life in the institution is much safer than in the outside world. The last tactic is the "conversation tactic" where the internee seems to accept the official interpretation and tries to play the role of the perfect internee, always showing enthusiasm for the institution.

When old people are admitted to institutions, they receive a folder with a number and a cover sheet. This contains information that will help identify the individual in the event of intercurrences or any legal or family issues. The information contained in the folders is cold and has no content that could provide more information about the subject's life story, which could give new contours to the institutional life of the characters who are part of this disturbing social context.

According to Miranda (2017), for Goffman (2008/2015), institutions fulfill the functions of integration and regulation through which individuals internalize a social order, in which interaction brings with it its own laws.

When you enter an institution for the elderly, you take practically nothing material with you, just some clothes, documents, small items of sentimental value linked to the individual's memories and portraits of the family and life in their youth.

The sudden change in social status is characterized by the removal of movable and immovable property, which is then managed by a relative, curator or caregiver responsible for the individual's care. Material goods and objects are part of the individual's life story. Without their belongings, individuals are stripped of their personalities and their established power, in many cases by amassing large sums of money that could support their old age outside the walls of a total institution. These aspects of detachment from belongings and objects seem to contribute to the strengthening of a new history of life and death without the glow of achievements.

Another very execrable fact brought about by the customs of a total institution of old people is characterized by the unveiling of intimate matters or hidden or negative facts brought about by that individual's personal life experience and which, upon entering the institution, are disseminated as "gossip" and "futricas" of interest to the institution's subordinates and service providers, in order to bring mediocre novelty to the context of that institution's daily life.

Another contamination inherent in the environment of total institutions is brought about by the codenames of "old people" and "new people", causing the person to lose their identity and not recognize themselves as a subject with desires and rights.

Goffman (2015, pp.54-58) investigated the "system of secondary adjustments" operating in the institutional dynamics of total establishments. This system, which is also correlated to that of privileges, is made up of practices that do not directly challenge the management team, but allow inmates to obtain forbidden satisfactions or to achieve, by forbidden means, permitted satisfactions. These practices can be called various things in the local lingo: "knowing which whistle to blow", "pulling the strings", "connivances", "trysts", etc.

The place where this system develops best is usually in prison, but it also appears in other total institutions.

Let's look again at Goffman (2015), who in his book deals with adaptive strategies to the environmental conditions of the total institution (GOFFMAN, 2015, pp.58-63). The inmate needs to adapt to the processes of admission, mortification and the system of privileges. This adaptation can take place in various ways and the inmate will employ different adaptive tactics throughout their "moral career", and can also switch between various strategies used as adaptive resources.

Some of these resources seem to be part of the universe of total institutions for the elderly:

Detachment from reality. This process of detachment can be seen as regression, depersonalization or alienation; intransigence can be translated as refusing to cooperate with the activities of daily life; colonization shows that the individual adapts to the establishment and ends up considering it a permanent home, believing that the place really represents the best of all worlds; conversation means accepting the role of the perfect inmate in order to follow the orders of the leaders and make them believe in the principles of the institution and its rules.

According to Goffman (2015), total institutions produce in their inmates a characteristic type and level of personal concern. "The internee is placed in an inferior social position compared to the one he occupied in the outside world, under the action of the processes of mortification and stripping to which he is subjected." (GOFFMAN, 2015, pp.63-69). As Goffman (2015) puts it, this sense of inferiority makes the behaviour of the institutionalized old person accommodating to the state of affairs that governs the behaviour, routine and norms imposed by the institutions through their leaders. In general, total institutions function as a depository for individuals, but they present themselves to society as efficient organizations, with effective work plans and technically perfect for the smooth running of the service offered to the institutionalized.

The management team must take into account the inmate's status and social relations in the outside world. According to Goffman (2015), inmates usually have a status and relations in the outside world and the institutional establishment needs to respect some of the inmates' rights as persons (GOFFMAN, 2015, p.71). The bureaucratic paperwork that requires the interdiction of an individual admitted to a psychiatric hospital and the transfer of their rights and duties to the guardianship of another person, who becomes their guardian and legal representative, has to be dealt with. The internee's eventual relations with society need to be managed: social security benefits, income tax, property maintenance, insurance, pensions, outstanding bills, etc.

It's worth noting that social roles are very evident in so-called institutional ceremonies, where leaders dress up, make speeches and welcome families and visitors as a great act of celebration. The "institutional ceremonies" tend to take place at certain intervals, arouse some social excitement, and all the groups in the establishment take part regardless of rank or position, but are given a place that expresses their position. A society dangerously divided between internees and management can be united through such ceremonies.

For Miranda (2017) "power is not an institution". This is the assertion that I think will be a crucial feature in the distinctions between Goffman's debate and Foucault's reflections. Despite some attempts to bring the two closer together, on account of the phenomenon of asylums or even through the idea of a modern society characterized by the spaces of enclosure, Foucault (2001) never intended to produce a kind of history of prisons or asylums, or even an impulse towards an analysis of prisons as a total institution.

> It's been said that I was trying to do the same thing as Erving Goffman in his work on asylums [...]. I'm not trying to do the same thing as Goffman. He is interested in the functioning of a certain type of institution: the total institution - asylum, school, prison. For my part, I try to show and analyze the relationship that exists between a set of power techniques and political forms such as the State. (FOUCAULT, 2001, p. 804).

For all the above reasons, it is essential nowadays to reflect on the process of confining people, which is characteristic of total institutions. A confinement that restricts, but does not imprison. It oppresses, but does not punish. It imposes rules, but does not dictate orders, through micro-relations of power.

Next, we'll look at the rules imposed by total institutions, as well as the subtle detachment of the identity of old people who have been confined.

3.4.Framing the Self and stripping away the identity case

We will begin this section by referring to the book "Surveillance and Punishment: The History of Violence in Prisons". In this book, Foucault (1975/2005) deals with the forms of violence practiced in prisons. In his study, the author develops modes of control with the aim of maintaining collective organization. During this process, Foucault also discusses the construction of disciplinary institutions. In the book, Foucault (2005) argues that although the institutions differ in their functionality, they share the same disciplinary forms, using ordering techniques and training practices.

It is important to point out that, in his "Microphysics of Power", Foucault (1979/2002) highlights the place where techniques are appropriated by bodies. Foucault demonstrates the body as a place of control in the imposition of adaptation and conformity through the exercise of power. For Foucault, power moves and inserts itself into bodies, making them objects and instruments in the economy of power, thus called disciplinary devices.

According to Foucault (2002), the aim of disciplinary devices is to obtain docile and useful bodies, i.e. bodies that are trained and prepared to behave in a way that suits and obeys the political interests of each social group.

According to Danner (2010) there is no theory of power in Foucault (1979). Foucault proposes an 'analytic of power'. There is no such thing as 'Power'; what exists are power relations, i.e. "disparate, heterogeneous forms, in constant transformation. Power is not a natural object, a thing; it is a social practice and, as such, historically constituted" (DANNER, 2010, p. 3).

What seems evident in Foucault's research (1979/2002) is the existence of a network of micro-powers articulated to the state and which run through the entire social structure. Therefore, it is exercised at lower levels of society, because it is not the state that uses micro-powers, but an articulated network of powers that manifests itself.

According to Foucault (1979):

> It's about [...] capturing power at its extremities, where it becomes capillary; capturing power in its most regional and local forms and institutions, especially at the point where, going beyond the rules of law that organize and delimit it, it extends itself, penetrates institutions, embodies itself in techniques and equips itself with instruments of material intervention, possibly violent ones (FOUCAULT, 1979, p. 182).

For Danner (2010), Foucault (1979) does not want to deny the importance of the state; his intention is to show that power relations go beyond the state level and extend throughout society. Let's put it this way: in modern times, it was not only the state that was the center of control and the formation of sociability; institutions such as the school, the sciences, the factory, the barracks, the hospice, etc. were also involved.

Still according to Danner (2010), the power worked on by Foucault (1979) is not a thing, a property that belongs to someone or some class; there are not, on the one hand, those who hold power (dominant) and, on the other, those who are subjected to it (dominated). In reality, 'Power' does not exist. Rather, there are practices or relations of power. Therefore, power is something that is exercised, that takes place, that works in a network and that must therefore be understood as a tactic, maneuver or strategy rather than a thing, an object or a good. In "Surveillance and Punishment", Foucault (1975) states:

Now, the study of this micro-physics presupposes that the power exercised within it is not conceived as a property, but as a strategy, that its effects of domination are not attributed to 'appropriation', but to dispositions, maneuvers, tactics, techniques, workings; that it reveals a network of relations that are always tense, always in activity, rather than a privilege that could be held; that it is the perpetual battle that is given as a model, rather than the contract that makes a cessation or a conquest that seizes a domain. In short, we have to admit that this power is exercised more than it is possessed, that it is not the acquired or preserved 'privilege' of the dominant class, but the overall effect of its strategic positions - an effect manifested and sometimes brought back by the position of those who are dominated. (FOUCAULT, 1975)

Danner (2010) analyzes Foucault's (1975) research and says that the author relates power to a kind of "functionality" of power. That is, the idea that power functions as a machinery that is not located in a specific place, but spreads throughout the social structure and permeates it. These are power relations that constitute a system of power, based on institutions that maintain a social, political link between them, based on the state, such as the state apparatus, the media, schools, factories, and what is legitimate and/or illegitimate to them as a common link in their relations (DANNER, 2010, p. 5).

An important aspect of Foucault's (1979) analysis of power (apud DANNER, 2010, p. 4) is the adoption of the model of war to make power relations intelligible. Thus, "power is war, war prolonged by other means". In other words, power is struggle, confrontation, dispute, power relations, strategy, where the aim is to accumulate advantages and multiply benefits. Therefore, it is in terms of war that we can best understand the way in which the extensive network of powers that runs through the social body unfolds and is articulated. (DANNER, 2010, p. 4).

When we think about the framing of the Self, we have to think about the techniques of power that Foucault (1975) calls disciplines. For Danner (2010), disciplines are techniques, mechanisms, devices of power, they are "methods that allow for the meticulous control of the body's operations, and which ensure the constant subjection of its forces and impose on it a relationship of docility-utility" (FOUCAULT, 1975, p. 129 apud DANNER, 2010, p. 8). In the text, Danner (2010) describes that disciplines work directly on individuals' bodies, manipulate their gestures and behavior, form them, train them (DANNER, 2010, p. 8).

Again using the concepts of Foucault (2004), in "The Hermeneutics of the Subject", the author discusses the devices of surveillance and social punishment in great depth. Surveillance and punishment devices are the means, forms and ways in which power is exercised in society. Disciplinary devices, on the other hand, are the mechanisms used discreetly to give force to the means that, if they aim at a certain end (FOUCAULT, 2004 apud BRIGIDO, 2013, pp. 62-64).

For Brigido (2013), the first disciplinary device used by society, according to Foucault (2004), is surveillance. Foucault also describes the strong surveillance power that exists in prisons, rehabilitation clinics, hospitals, in short, in the way that places where human beings are treated are built and structured. However, in order to be more precise about the effectiveness of surveillance, the philosophy of control by looking was created. The figure of the inspector was born (FOUCAULT, 2004).

Still for Brigido (2013), Foucault (2004) says that the application of punishment becomes a bureaucratic procedure, allowing punishment to be made official by the state, but, at the same time, for justice or the state system to take a certain distance from the practice of punishment. This distance justifies the acts of punishment. "Such acts are presented as necessary to correct, re-educate and cure those who are violators of law and order. It is the institutionalization of the right to punish" (BRIGIDO, 2013, p. 63).

Brigido (2013) says that Foucault (2004) analyzes other systems of punishment, but focuses his analysis on prison, because the prison system makes the exercise of punishment natural and legitimate, "it puts an end to the exaggerations of punishment, but it gives legality to disciplinary mechanisms. When punishment becomes "legal", it can be inflicted by power without being seen as excessive. The power to punish becomes discreet" (BRIGIDO, 2013, p. 63).

Foucault's (2004) theories on adjusting behavior and disciplinary rules lead us to think about how contemporary society views aging and the ways in which power is exercised over old age. Since old age is a process of loss, it seems obvious to us that the disciplinary devices developed by Foucault become naturalized in the light of a capitalist society that uses technological resources in health to prolong decrepit old age or to submit the elderly to a space of confinement that proclaims peace, tranquillity, norms and processes of care, coated in rules, impositions and sublimation of desires.

Contextualizing the production of stereotypes built to highlight the aging body and its natural losses in the process of senescence, which individuals go through until their complete degeneration, makes us imagine how much the marginalization of aging, the exclusion and concealment of old age produce suffering. The old person becomes a prisoner of institutional rules, capable of promoting the existential annihilation of aging individuals who lack affection and attention. The subjugation of rules in this oppressive context of disciplinary institutions is not part of youthfulness, active engagement, self-confidence and the new social representation of old age today.

'Getting sick and failing'. This is the discourse disseminated by the new social order of successful old age[9] .

In 2005, the Brazilian government released a document from the *World Health Organization* called "Active aging: a health policy". The document's introduction recommends the following:

The ageing of the population raises several fundamental questions for policymakers.

---

9 "Recognizing the plurality of aging experiences does not imply that dependence is not the natural condition of those who grow old, nor does it propose that there are no limits to cultural and technological investment in biological processes. Successful and innovative ageing cannot close the door on abandoned and dependent old age, nor turn it into a consequence of personal neglect (...) In a context in which unemployment and underemployment affect ever larger contingents of the younger population, the costs involved in old age, especially those involved in the later stages of life, are growing in the same proportion as the technological advances put into action to prolong human life". (DEBERT, 1997).

> How can we help people remain independent and active as they age? How can we encourage health promotion and prevention policies, especially those aimed at older people? As people are living longer, how can the quality of life in old age be improved? Will a large number of people in old age cause our health and social security systems to fail? How can we balance the role of the family and the state in terms of assisting those who need care as they age? How can we recognize and support the important role that older people play in caring for others? (WORLD HEALTH ORGANIZATION, 2005, p.7).

The document addressed a series of concerns. "Its target audience includes government officials at all levels, non-governmental entities and the private sector, and all those responsible for formulating policies and programs linked to ageing" (BRASIL, 2005, p.7). The document aims to approach the issue of health from a broad perspective and even recognizes the fact that health needs an intersectoral approach. "It also suggests that health professionals lead the project if we really want healthy older people to continue to represent a resource for their families, communities and economies" (BRASIL, 2005, p.7), according to the WHO Declaration on Ageing and Health, in Brasilia in 1996.

The first part of this document describes the worldwide growth of the population over 60, especially in developing countries.

The second part explores the concept and foundation of "active aging" as a goal for the formulation of policies and programs.

The third part summarizes the evidence on the factors that determine whether or not individuals and populations can have a positive quality of life as they age.

The final part of the document, part four, discusses seven important challenges associated with an ageing population for governments and the non-governmental, academic and private sectors.

The fifth part of the document "provides an action plan for active ageing and concrete suggestions for key action proposals". It proposes that the "action plan and suggestions are intended to serve as a basis for the development of more specific local, regional and national actions, in line with the action plan adopted by the Second United Nations World Assembly on Ageing in 2002". (WORLD HEALTH ORGANIZATION, 2005, p.7).

When we analyze the entire content of the document drawn up by the UN, we see the clear concern about the repercussions that the advent of aging could have on the productive system. In view of this disturbing context, forms and strategies have been devised to outline a form of aging that denotes a sense of success in the process of growing old, but which is still anchored to the dogmas of capital, with a view to using means that promote the accumulation of wealth by old individuals. The aim is to ensure that these individuals continue to produce well into old age, maintained by health technologies and biomedicine, at the service of innovations that maximize the functional capacity of those who place the success of their lives in longevity.

With the advance of health technologies, biomedicine implements in its practices the concept that if the subject falls ill, it is because he or she has failed to comply with the rules adopted by the protocols of health well-being, strategies of what Foucault (1975) called biopolitics. Therefore, the sick person is to blame for the failure of self-care. As far as ageing is concerned, we understand that decrepit old age finds no space in socially considered healthy environments and therefore suffers from the same evils as the punishment imposed by the rules of self-care. As a result, due to the imposition of social rules, the ageing must be removed to closed institutions to accommodate the symptoms of sadness, loneliness and forgetfulness.

According to Farhi Neto (2007), the term 'biopolitics' appeared publicly for the first time, to our knowledge, in a series of lectures given by Foucault on social medicine in 1974, in Rio de Janeiro. Still according to Farhi Neto (2007), the three conferences in Rio, in October 1974, mark a moment in the history of Foucault's work.

that Foucault's analytical point of view begins to shift in relation to Surveillance and Punishment, moving away from the strict plane of a microphysics, proper to the analysis of institutions such as the prison, the asylum or the hospital, and becoming interested in the plane of the microphysics of power, in which the word 'politics' refers to the way in which the State seeks to guide relations of power.

> [...] The theory of sovereignty presupposes the subject: it aims to ground the essential unity of power and is always developed in a preliminary element of the law. Threefold "primitivism", then: that of the subject who must be subjected, that of the unity of power that must be founded and that of the legitimacy that must be respected. Subject, unity of power and law: these are the elements between which the theory of sovereignty operates. (FOUCAULT, 1999, P. 50)

Interpreting Foucault, I believe that biopower translates into the organization of the state, which establishes control over individuals' obligations to the law and to the government in exchange for protection, health and other components that guarantee social rights. Its reach and effectiveness over lives lies in managing power relations directed at a population mass, the survival of the collective of peoples and nations.

For Foucault, the state's guarantee of human rights makes individuals citizens, and citizens have rights and obligations towards the state, subjugating individuals to docile bodies, so that the state can intervene on these individuals through relations of power.

While biopolitics focuses on populations, especially the long-term effects of population ageing in the different nations of the world, the framing of ageing subjects, on the other hand, are procedures, rooted in the culture of disciplinary institutions. It is up to these closed institutions to maintain the imperative of the rules established to preserve life.

3.5. Old age in the documentary "Come Sweet Death"

The documentary "Come Sweet Death" was made in 1967 and directed by Sergio Bernardes Filho. The director was the son of the famous architect of the same name, Sergio Bernardes (also known as Sergio Bernardes Filho), and was born in 1944 in Rio de Janeiro. In 1962, he began his film studies at IDHEC *(Institute des Hautes Etudes Cinematographiques)* in Paris. Then, still in Europe, he studied choreography and theater with Maurice Bejart and composed the soundtrack with musician Pierre Henry. He returned to Brazil in the second half of the 1960s and made two films, the short documentary "Come Sweet Death" (1967), about the Sao Luiz asylum (RJ), and the feature-length fiction "Desperate" (1968), which unanimously won Best Film, Best Actor (Raul Cortez) and Best Actress (Marisa Urban) at the 1968 Belo Horizonte Film Festival[10] .

The movie.

The scene opens with one of the religious nuns who ran the asylum at the time describing the daily routine of the old people institutionalized in the Asylum. The first

10 See: http://www.heco.com.br/colecoes-de-dvds?ID=68

scene of the movie shows one of the old people's meals and then the same old people are seen at morning mass.

In his research, Groisman (1999a) portrays the construction of the universe of asylums and describes some of the history of the creation of the Sao Luiz Asylum for Destitute Old People.

Groisman (1999a) reports that when they arrived in Brazil in 1890, the French nuns belonging to the Little Family of the Sacred Heart of Jesus (based in Allois, France) were welcomed by the church. Imbued with the purpose of building the Asilo Sao Luiz, Viscount Ferreira de Almeida, the founder of the institution, invited the nuns to join him in managing the work.

Groisman (1999a) describes in his research that the emergence of the Asilo Sao Luiz is indissolubly linked to the figure of its founder, but for Groisman there is no relevance in the emergence of the Asilo through its founder, but rather as a consequence of the historical and social context of that time, related to the social construction of old age as an age category and the very practice of philanthropy, exercised through assistance to old age.

Returning to the documentary, in the next scene we see the nun presenting the routine of the elderly in the film. She tells the viewer that right after breakfast, the old people go out into the yard to play with the birds and sing songs.

But who are the old people at the Sao Luiz Asylum for Destitute Old People at the beginning of the 20th century?

According to Groisman (1999a), the old people taken in by the asylum were of both sexes, without distinction of color or nationality, probably destitute, to whom the São Luiz shelter provided a home, food, clothing, a doctor and a pharmacy, and for the dead, a modest but decent burial.

It is curious to observe the image of old age at the beginning of the 20th century in the city of Rio de Janeiro. According to Groisman (1999a) in his research:

On Sunday, the day was beautiful, clear and cheerful. I set out to go to Caju beach, the place where several cemeteries are gathered. (...) The streetcar runs lightly through this corner of the city. Caju beach is a place full of contrasts that make a vivid impression. On one side, the cemetery, with its apparent expression of death: on the other, the sea, the bay, where the speedboats whistle, the ferries pass quickly, the ships unload and receive cargo. On the one hand, the appearance of paralysis and death, on the other, the intense life, the constant bustle. A perfect contrast[11] .

The documentary "Come Sweet Death" resumes its scene and, at this moment, we see the elderly reminiscing, telling their life stories and trying to hold on to their social representations before institutionalization. For a moment, the scene of reminiscing is interrupted so that the nun can inform the viewer that the elderly will retire for the evening.

In his research, Groisman (1999a) deals with the "shipwrecked of life". At the beginning of the 20th century, social assistance was a very complicated field. At the same time as philanthropic institutions were flourishing, the population had very ambivalent feelings about urban poverty. It was necessary to define those who really deserved and should be assisted according to criteria aimed at preserving order and combating idleness and the "vices" that characterized vagrancy.

Still according to Groisman (1999a), this dichotomy between good and bad elements, between those who would be supported and those who would be repressed seems to be one of the aspects that influenced the formation of images of old age in care.

Returning to the documentary, the nun informs the viewer that at 2:30 p.m. the elderly return to the chapel to pray the tergo aloud and at 4:00 p.m. they start dinner. At 17:30 they pray the tergo again. Suddenly, the scene changes and a wing appears with other elderly people who live at the Asilo Sao Luiz para Velhice Desamparada. The space I'm referring to is called *PAVILLON SAINT LOUIS. Societe Franqaise de Bienfaisance de* Rio de Janeiro. I had the opportunity to get to know this space up close, because from August 2017 to March 2018, I was hired to run the institution. This institution, which cohabits the same geographical space as the Sao Luiz Asylum for destitute old people, is a French Benevolent Society, now called *Residence Huguette Fraga,* which, by tradition of the culture of that country, came to Brazil to provide social assistance to communities of children in a region of poverty in the city of Rio de Janeiro and also to welcome French elderly people who came to Brazil at a young age and who receive old-age benefits from the French government. I won't go

11 "Na ponte do Caju - o Asylo Sao Luis" - Jornal do Brasil, Rio de Janeiro, 1908.

into the routine of the *Huguette Fraga Residence* because, like any closed institution, it suffers the same influence as the aspects of confinement described so far about total institutions. Let's go back to the documentary "Come Sweet Death".

The nun who introduces the documentary appears again to inform the viewer that at 7pm everyone goes to sleep "in the hope that the next day will come". Following the scene, another much older nun appears and discusses the concept of death. She talks about the divine laws of finitude and that no individual can escape them. The scene continues with the arrival of a hearse carrying a priest. The nun makes a point of showing the morgue where the docile bodies are waiting for the final judgment. From this scene onwards, the film shows the preparations for the removal of yet another aged body that lived out its last days in that place. The film depicts the removal of the old corpse while the elderly living dead say goodbye to this body mortified by institutional life and the failure of its organ functions. It's interesting to note that the director of the film brings the scene of the hearse driving away from the asylum as a representation of the farewell of the old friends who will also one day say goodbye to that place in the same way. All the old people make their way to the car to say their final goodbyes to that mortified, forgotten and inert body in the last moments of its life. The last scene of the film features a circus made up of all the nuns of the institution celebrating the service they have offered and the fulfillment of their religious duty towards those who sought the proper reception in the institution until their physical death.

In the text, Groisman (1999a) refers to "the place of old age and old age as a place". For Groisman (1999a, p. 104), the newspaper reports seem to make it clear that old age had gained a "place" in the city. Located on the Caju bridge, the Sao Luiz asylum was this "home" for the elderly. However, the "location" of old age was not only geographical, but also symbolic. In this sense, the asylum was seen as a kind of "limbo", where old age was outside of time and space: sacralized, it was between heaven and earth; seen as degeneracy, between life and death; alienated from the world, between the past and the present... With the emergence of the asylum, old age gained a "place", but at the same time symbolically lost its place in life. Old people were expected to do nothing but wait for death.

3.6. The world of the internee and the tactics of withdrawal and conversation

We will begin our journey in the world of institutions for the elderly, based on a discussion of the inmate who lives in these institutions and the behaviours and consequences that characterize the inmate and his world with imaginary borders and the conversions necessary for the disciplinary power of closed institutions, with the aim of perfect social control and the exemplary maintenance of institutional rules to better preserve the *status quo*.

Let's go back to Foucault. According to Foucault (1987),

> Discipline sometimes requires a fence, the specification of a place that is heterogeneous to all others and closed in on itself.
>
> A place protected from disciplinary monotony. There was the great "incarceration" of vagrants and the miserable; there were others that were more discreet, but insidious and efficient (FOUCAULT, 1987, p. p.168).

In order to better understand Foucault's (1987) thinking on disciplinary and normative conduct, we turn to a reflection that is relevant to the context of our research. Foucault (1987) uses the concepts of tactics, the spatial ordering of men; taxonomy, the disciplinary space of natural beings; the economic framework, the regulated movement of wealth (FOUCAULT, 1987, p. 175).

In order to better contextualize asylum spaces, we will highlight a very appropriate definition of Foucault's theories (1987), taxonomy and tactics. For Foucault (1987), the function of taxonomy is to characterize (and therefore reduce) individual singularities. While natural taxonomy is situated on the axis from character to category, disciplinary tactics is situated on the axis linking the singular and the multiple. It allows for both the characterization of the individual as an individual and the ordering of a given multiplicity. It is the primary condition for the control and use of a set of distinct elements: the basis for a microphysics of power that Foucault called a "cell".

It is worth reflecting on the tactics so well outlined by Foucault (1987) in a shelter for the elderly. In nursing homes, care procedures take precedence over the other rules established in disciplinary institutions. The elderly person in the asylum represents an 'object' to be cared for. When they enter nursing homes, they don't seem to realize that elements built up over a lifetime will be left behind in exchange for care related to the routine maintenance of daily life.

Institutionalized elderly people are presented with a routine of care without the innovations necessary for the dynamics of human life. In nursing homes, there is a reproduction of procedures that lead caregivers into alienation without the proper questioning of what they are doing and why they are doing it. The inmate in a nursing home has no options in the day-to-day life of the institution, making the need for food and the execution of care and hygiene procedures fundamental to the existence of institutionalized individuals.

In order to better understand the control tactics exercised by the institutions of old age, we resorted to an analogy with the theories of Foucault (1987) regarding subliminal power tactics and the resources for good training.

In the tactics of power so well treated by Foucault (1987), we see that constituted power is transmuted into invisible power, largely instituted by bureaucratic norms. The power implicit in nursing home institutions accompanies the history of the institution as well as its dogmas, beliefs and the conjuncture through which the social institution was built to characterize the social reputation of the society in which it originated.

According to Foucault (1987), disciplinary power is, in fact, a power which, instead of appropriating and withdrawing, has the main function of "training"; or without a doubt, training in order to withdraw and appropriate even more and better. It doesn't bind forces in order to reduce them; it tries to connect them in order to multiply them and use them as a whole. Discipline "manufactures" individuals; it is the specific technique of a power that takes individuals both as objects and as instruments of its exercise (FOUCAULT. 1987, p.195).

In nursing homes, the atmosphere of distancing the subject from their stories, their desires, their belongings and their impulses, can lead to 'repressive' impulses that remove painful conflicts and frustrations from consciousness to be experienced and remembered, repressing or repressing them into the unconscious, making them unpleasant and forgettable[12] .

---

12 Fungencio (2008) says that "Repression, in Freud's view, is a psychic defense

The sensation felt in the institutional environments of old people about the processes of conversion to the rules of the institution imposed on a supposed coexistence in nursing homes, come adapted from very conservative and castrating rules, which are based on obsolete norms, but which are imperative to the results related to the daily care of human life.

Returning to the film "The Exterminating Angel", we will next find ourselves analyzing scene two, where we will have the opportunity to revisit an analogy pertinent to the universe of closed institutions and the aspects of imprisonment and suffocation of subjects in their desires.

3.7. Movie "The Exterminating Angel" - take - scene two (The lockdown)

During the dinner scene, the guests in the living room listen to music and maintain the exemplary behavior characteristic of bourgeois customs. As the hours go by, the characters in the movie feel that something strange is going on in the room. They realize that there is no way out, no way to leave the place. The atmosphere of confinement is surreal because there is no logic to explain why the characters can't get out of the mansion that houses them. The characters will have to test their limits, impulses and resistance. The foundation of Bunuel's film, an atypical space-time relationship, mediated by the psychological and social dimensions of the characters, is put to the test when everyone is caught up in their own "web" of meanings. Intrigues between the guests, lies and extramarital affairs are unraveled by the sense of imminent imprisonment characteristic of confinement.

As dawn breaks in the mansion, the confinement seems to penetrate the guts of each character. Accommodation to that state of affairs is questionable, but everyone initially seems to accept the rules established by the lockdown. As the scene continues, there is a slight strangeness in the characters, as there is an attempt to resist what is being imposed on the guests of the mansion, in the Foucauldian sense, as a potential for revolt, the ability to rebel and insurgent through

---

procedure used by the organism to get rid of stimuli or excitations that cause displeasure. Without the possibility of escaping (by motor action) or eliminating (by satisfaction or discharge) certain excitations that cause displeasure, our psyche tries to eliminate them by removing them from the quality of being conscious" (FUNGENCIO, 2008, p. 238 .

different ways of acting (MAIA, 1995), but soon afterwards, the attempt at resistance is replaced by the accommodation of those individuals. One of the guests rebels against the state of affairs portrayed in that chaotic environment.

Slowly, imprisonment awakens primitive instincts among the film's subjects. When the scarcity of food and water becomes a reality, the drive to survive brings new conflicts to the human relationships established in that mansion. The characters try to mitigate the imprisonment, but it becomes overwhelming, totalitarian and inhuman towards those subjects who find themselves fragile to the impositions suffered by the power structures. During the imprisonment scene, a sense of disorientation in time and space arises, characteristic of the process of confinement, leading some of the characters to delirium. In the struggle against confinement, feelings of enclosure, resistance or accommodation are being put to the test so that the subjects can re-signify their desires beyond resistance (Freudian and Foucauldian) and conformism in adapting to norms, rules, dogmas, ideologies, conversation and social annihilation.

The next chapter will look at the malaise of growing old in contemporary culture and the implications for the institutionalization of old age. Subjective and socio-cultural dimensions will be confronted, using concepts from Freud and Foucault, ending with an analysis of a film production.

4. MAL ESTAR NAS ILPIS - BACK AND FORTH

This chapter sought to reflect theoretically on the discomfort of growing old in contemporary times and to think about existing in old age, especially emphasizing the circumstances of institutionalization of old people, when desire has no room for expression or forms of sublimation, a time when disciplinary institutions use their tactics and strategies to maintain docile bodies that are manageable to the controls in place. In this sense, reflections are made on care and the practice of self, seeking to verify the ways of resisting and producing and preserving social memory, through reminiscences that give new meaning to existence in the advanced age.

4.1. The discomfort of growing old in contemporary times

According to Campos (2001), the interpretation of culture is one of the most traditional "applied" themes in psychoanalysis. Campos comments in his article that one cannot fail to notice the reinforcement that psychoanalytic interpretations of culture have gained. For the author, this is mainly due to a series of questions posed by the socio-historical context of contemporaneity. Campos (2007) states that the exploitation of violence, new forms of psychic suffering, the biologization of the social[13] and the crisis of psychoanalysis are at the heart of the concerns at the beginning of the 21st century.

Using Joel Birman (2001), we identify that the thinker delves into the complexity of reflecting on the knowledge, ideologies and practices that define

---

13 "The last decade has seen the biologism of a new "natural science" creep wolfishly into academic discourse, which increasingly mirrors the legacy of the ludic and "post-sociological" fashion of deconstructivism. At first glance, it seemed that genetic research would be able to debunk racist nonsense with scientific arguments. Researchers such as Swedish molecular geneticist Svante Paabo have proven that men from the most diverse nations, by virtue of their DNA sequences, can be genetically more "related" to each other than to their half-wall neighbors. But these findings are now increasingly under the weight of a new "biologization" of social conduct, for which, incidentally, the geneticists themselves are ready to provide the ammunition (...) Such scholars are often naïve from a social point of view and thus perhaps don't realize how their "purely objective" research is influenced by ideological currents that undermine society. It goes without saying that the reduction of human culture and sociability to the standard of molecular biology provides arguments for the legitimization of a renewed barbarism" (KURTZ, 1996).

malaise in contemporary times.

Campos (2007), when analyzing Birman's (2001) proposal, states that the author starts from a genuinely Freudian position on the Psychoanalysis and Culture interface, believing that it is in analyzing the limits and impasses of these two fields that a mutual contribution can be achieved (BIRMAN, 2001 apud CAMPOS, 2007).

Campos (2007) states that Birman (2001) starts from the fundamental work on the psychoanalytic interpretation of culture, "Malaise in Civilization" (FREUD, 1929), putting it into perspective with contemporary malaise, through a Foucauldian analytical framework.

The question posed by Campos (2007) is: if Freud analyzed and described the characteristics of the malaise inherent in the tragic condition of the modern subject, what would be the status of the question today?

In "The Malaise of Civilization", Freud (1929) presents the thesis that culture produces a malaise in human beings, since there is an insurmountable antagonism between the demands of the drive and those of civilization. Thus, for the good of society, the individual is sacrificed: in order for civilization to develop, man has to pay the price of renouncing drive satisfaction (man's sex life and aggressiveness are severely damaged).

For Lima (2007), Freud (1930) points out that every individual is an enemy of civilization, since all men have destructive, antisocial and anti-cultural tendencies. Civilization, therefore, wages a constant struggle against isolated man and his freedom, replacing the power of the individual with the power of the community. Human suffering comes from three main factors: the body, the external world and relationships (FREUD, 1930 apud LIMA, 2007).

In his text, Freud (1930) points to some of the methods that exist in human society to avoid suffering and seek happiness (even if only partial). Among these methods, he mentions the use of drugs, the sublimation of impulses, work, fantasies, delusional remodeling, love and neurotic illness (symptoms are substitute satisfactions for unfulfilled desires) (FREUD, 1930).

For Freud (1930), there is a close relationship between civilization and the feeling of guilt. Civilization only achieves its goal of keeping human beings connected by increasingly strengthening the feeling of guilt, developing a superego whose influence produces cultural evolution (FREUD, 1930).

Returning to the question posed by Campos (2007). When he describes the characteristics of the malaise inherent in the tragic condition of the modern subject, what would be the status of the question today?

From this questioning, we want to refer to the malaise of aging in contemporary times, because according to estimates by the World Health Organization (WHO, 2014 apud MOREIRA and NOGUEIRA, 2008), the population of people over 60 makes up a total of 600 million elderly people, and will increase from the current 841 million to 2 billion by 2050[14] .

For Moreira and Nogueira (2008), Brazil, once referred to as a country of young people, has also been making its demographic transition and is undergoing a rapid process of population ageing, a fact attributed to the two factors already mentioned: increased life expectancy and reduced birth rates. It is predicted that by 2020, of the 1.2 billion elderly people in the world, 34 million Brazilians will be over the age of 60, which will correspond to the sixth oldest population on the planet (MINAYO; COIMBRA JUNIOR, 2002 apud MOREIRA and NOGUEIRA, 2008).

According to Moreira and Nogueira (2008), population ageing is taking place in the midst of profound economic, social, political, ideological and scientific transformations. Living and growing old in this scenario of instability, marked by rapid changes in knowledge and cultural values, characterized by the phenomenon of 14 globalization and consumerism, which results in the rapid obsolescence of objects, people and relationships, is an experience that generates insecurity and unease for the contemporary subject.

For Moreira and Nogueira (2008), thinking about the contemporary experience of ageing certainly implies considering the intertwining of the socio-cultural environment in which this experience takes place with its historical determinants. In this context, there are countless occurrences - social, cultural, political and economic - which influence lifestyles, values and social patterns and, consequently, people's

---

See: www.who.int/hpr/ageing

ways of being and the psychic structures that are produced. Uncertainty, turbulence, continuous change, technological explosion and globalization constitute the present day and demand new and rapid responses on an individual and collective level.

Analyzing the aging process and its challenges in the face of the imperative issues of capitalism raises several questions. Why is it so difficult to accept the natural process of ageing? Why do social issues have a devastating impact on the pulses that accompany human nature throughout the process of existence?

For Moreira and Nogueira (2008), understanding this has been a challenge for researchers in various fields, and the divergence between the various theorists on the meanings of post-modernity or contemporaneity is evident. For Featherstone (1995), what is called post-modernity is not simply a theoretical formulation, but something that is also driven by artistic and cultural movements that refer to the changes we are experiencing today. According to this author, the terms post-modernity, post-modernism, post-modern and their derivatives were first used by Federico de Onis in the 1930s, but took off in the 1960s in the New York art scene, making inroads into the fields of architecture, music, literature and the human sciences.

Still according to Moreira and Nogueira (2008), post-modernity or contemporaneity can be defined from various points of view, but it will always be characterized by the emergence of a media culture in which the social scene is based on a strong appeal to consumption, stimulated by the mass media, which have contributed decisively to making the image sovereign, marking society by the phenomenon of the "aestheticization of everyday life" (FEATHERSTHONE, 1995). Beauty, youth, happiness, the perfect body and personal success are goods or commodities that can be purchased.

This aesthetic value advocated by the new anti-ageing technologies that have emerged within a media culture, imposes a feeling that individuals will no longer be able to age, causing a malaise in continuing the natural course of life inherent to all human beings on the planet.

With regard to some aspects imposed by contemporary society, in terms of the cultural values dictated by the ideologies of capital that youth, beauty and power should be predominant in the social behavior of aging individuals, Moreira and

Nogueira (2008) argue that these societies are markedly individualistic, narcissistic, exhibitionist and lacking in solidarity, and that aging is invested with negative values, making the old, old age and growing old something undesirable and generating suffering.

In order to characterize this malaise of ageing in contemporary society, it is worth highlighting once again the questions raised by Moreira and Nogueira (2008). The experience of ageing tends to be seen as an individual choice, a lifestyle in the face of a wide range of products and services, and no longer as an inevitable experience of the passing years. Aging is a struggle against old age itself, culminating in the adoption of manic practices that give the sensation of restoring lost youth, in the incessant quest to prevent the "inevitable".

Considering all the issues brought up in the reflection on "the malaise of aging in contemporary times", it is worth noting that all these aspects affect the institutionalized elderly more intensely, because these old individuals, incapable and forgotten by society, have nothing left but mechanisms of reminiscence and resistance. These mechanisms can guarantee that they can cope with the order imposed on the frail elderly, as a means of managing the effects of the pulse of life or the pulse of death, constructive or destructive forces that emerge throughout life and become more acute in late ageing.

4.2. Pulse of life and pulse of death in aging

A pulse is an impulse, inherent in organic life, to restore a previous state of affairs, an impulse that the living entity has been forced to abandon under pressure from external disturbing forces Freud (2005, p. 140)

According to Goldfarb (1997), in order to understand why people close to the age of 50 are considered old, we have to consider that, at the dawn of the 20th century, not only did life expectancy not exceed 50 or 55 years, but traditional pre-war society reserved the social role of old people for these people. And psychoanalysis still had a long way to go.

Around the age of 50, unfavorable conditions are created for psychoanalysis. The accumulation of psychic material makes the work more difficult, the time needed for recovery becomes too long and the possibilities for psychic processes to find new paths begin to stall (FREUD 1904, Volume II).

For Goldfarb (1997), the subject of psychoanalysis is a response to the anxieties of a divided, decentered "individual", dominated by an unconscious that speaks for him. This subject of desire is based on otherness, it anticipates the parental desire that determines it as subject to the desire of the other.

Goldfarb (1997) argues that the certainty of inhabiting a single body, always the same, whatever its modifications, is the guarantee of identity and permanence in the relationship with the other. To achieve this, the subject must give the same relational meaning to a series of experiences, even though they happened at different times, in other words, they must also have a temporal meaning.

Let's remember the episode that happened to Freud when he was 63:

I can tell you about a similar adventure that happened to me. I was sitting alone in my compartment of the sleeper car when, due to a violent bump in the train, the door leading to the adjoining bathroom opened and a man of a certain age, wearing a suit and a travel cap, entered my cabin. I imagined that when he came out of the bathroom between the two, he had taken a wrong turn and entered my compartment by mistake. I hurried to inform him of the mistake, but realized, completely perplexed, that the intruder was none other than my own image reflected in the mirror of the communication door. I also remember that this apparition deeply displeased me (FREUD, 1919, p. 57).

Reflecting on Freud's thoughts about himself and old age, we can consider that the losses inherent in aging fill us with anguish as we face the finitude and decrepitude characteristic of the process of life and death.

Regarding this perspective on growing old, Goldfarb (1997) argues that the old person is always the other in whom we don't recognize ourselves. The image of old age always seems to be "outside", on the other side, and although we know that "it" is our image, it produces an impression of disquieting strangeness, the terrifying linked to the familiar. Frightening because the mirror image no longer corresponds to the memory image; the mirror image anticipates or confirms old age, while the memory image wants to be an idealized image that refers to the familiarity of the specular Self.

This whole context leads us to conceptualize what Freud called the life drive and the death drive.

According to Goldfarb (1997), the concept of the Death Pulse, introduced in

"Beyond the Pleasure Principle" and constantly reaffirmed by Freud until the end of his work (and his life), will from then on represent one of the greatest controversies in the psychoanalytic field, which is definitively linked to the areas of philosophy and anthropology. This study addresses issues such as violence, aggression, ambivalence, sadism, masochism and repetition compulsion.

It is interesting to analyze that when we reflect on the pulse of life, it is charged with energetic exchanges. The death drive, on the other hand, becomes regressive. Therefore, the death drive in old age may be related to finitude, dementia and institutionalization. In the words of Goldfarb (1997):

> Being old can often mean losing the illusion of one's own potency, accepting the inescapable dominance of the death drive and, despite this, continuing to fight. It's a difficult struggle, because the mourning that has to be done is that of life itself, a mourning that acts by anticipation, mourning for an object that is still preserved, but condemned: and the threat of annihilation by death is not a feeling that anyone can adapt to. The "I", before anything else, demands continuity (GOLDFARB, 1997, p. 15).

But if old age is a process of thinking about the ruptures of narcissistic ideas, what makes old individuals accommodate themselves to their bodies and gradually surrender to the social rules that determine that old age should be subject to the sublimation of desires, attitudes and obedience?

4.3. The disciplinary institution and docile bodies in Foucault

When we look at Foucault's book **Surveillance and Punishment** (1987), it is inevitable that we will be struck by the disciplinary practices exercised in 18th century France, which make us think of the procedures used to punish the condemned, causing them pain and asking for forgiveness. This established the mechanisms of social control over individuals.

According to Billout (2003), in the 18th century, there was a cry among jurists and philosophers that even the worst of murderers should have their humanity respected in terms of punishment (BILLOUT, 2003 apud SOUZA; MENEZES, 2010).

The shift from punishment to the body establishes a new disciplinary rule for the mechanisms of power that were aimed at a kind of modulation of individual behavior. The new rules established allowed individuals to be monitored and at the same time imposed a disciplinary order.

Power over the body, on the other hand, did not completely cease to exist until the middle of the 19th century. Without a doubt, punishment was no longer centered on torment as a technique of suffering; it took as its object the loss of a good or a right. (FOUCAULT, 1987, p. 19)

Billouet (2003) points out that:

These mechanisms that intensify power and production differ from the functioning of real power, which blocked the intensity of counterforces. They appear at a time when disciplinary institutions are multiplying, schools and charitable institutions are making it possible to observe and control society in depth [...] (BILLOUET, 2003, p. 133).

On the history of prisons, Foucault (2005) shows that disciplinary modes and power regimes are structured not only in prisons, but also in schools, asylums, hospitals, barracks and why not say in society itself, where subtle mechanisms of surveillance and social control exercise and practice power, characterized by a norm produced according to the essence of each of these institutions.

According to Sousa and Meneses (2010), in Europe in the 17th century, internment became a movement for the seclusion and exclusion of individuals, with not only the insane being interned, but also the poor and those considered vagrants. The first disciplinary institutions were created, in which all those who were on the margins of society were imprisoned, and the insane were part of this group.

According to Souza and Meneses (2010), it is worth noting that at this time the Church allied itself with the State in favor of this new form of power. Thus, confinement symbolized the redemption of reprehensible morals and the enclosure of evil. Internment served as much to lock up the insane and punish vagrants as it did to console the poor. In this way, the church exercised power over the poor, the sick and the miserable who submitted to the mechanisms of power.

For Foucault (2005), punishment and surveillance are mechanisms of power used to docilize and train people to conform to the norms established in institutions. Surveillance is a technology of power that affects individuals' bodies, controlling their gestures, their activities, their learning and their daily lives. According to the author:

[...] Disciplinary power is [...] a power that, instead of appropriating and withdrawing, has the main function of "training": or, without a doubt, training in order to withdraw and appropriate even more and better. It doesn't bind the forces in order to reduce them; it tries to bind them in order to multiply them and use them as a whole. [...] It "trains" the confused multitudes [...] (FOUCAULT, 2005, p.143).

Reflecting on Foucault, how can we appropriate the study of disciplinary power today?

Sousa and Meneses (2010) argue that disciplinary power is the result of transformations in bourgeois society, the shift of sovereign power to the social body. From then on, power was exercised in the form of micro-powers or micro-politics. This power is exercised over individual bodies by means of exercises specifically aimed at increasing their strength. The aim of these exercises was to train and docilize bodies.

"It is a docile body that can be submitted to, that can be used, that can be transformed and perfected" (FOUCAULT, 2005, p.118).

It's interesting to think that discipline exercises a kind of distribution of individuals into spaces, using rules and norms of incarceration and enclosure for this purpose.

But Foucault's point about power over bodies is worth highlighting. This body will only be useful if it is productive or submissive. This subjection constitutes what Foucault (2005) calls the microphysics of power.

The author talks about this microphysics of power:

[...] a multiplicity of often minimal processes, of different origins, sparsely located, which [...] circulated sometimes very quickly (between the army and technical schools or colleges and high schools), sometimes slowly and more discreetly (insidious militarization of large workshops) [...] (FOUCAULT, 2005, p. 119).

For Souza and Meneses (2010), disciplinary practices allow the control of the operations of bodies and the constant subjection of their strength, imposing on them a relationship of docility and usefulness. The authors also discuss one of the main characteristics of disciplinary power and the attention paid by disciplines to the distribution of individuals within a space.

According to Foucault (2005), disciplinary procedures become increasingly meticulous. From then on, discipline will determine the individual's distribution in space by means of techniques such as the principle of enclosure and the queue. These techniques are applied in schools, barracks, hospitals and factories, making it possible to observe and monitor individuals in the physical space in which they are located. In this way, enclosure facilitates the system of surveillance and control between individuals.

"Enclosure" consists of establishing organization in physical space. In a nursing home, for example, there are bedrooms and rooms for certain activities such as watching TV, eating meals or doing nothing. An identification form for this elderly inmate will indicate their entry into the institution and their habits and behavior in the face of institutionalization. A series of details locate the individual in the nursing home: carers, monitoring cameras, a guard at the entrance door and maintenance staff, characterizing a kind of surveillance of the individual without the individual being aware of the control without looking.

Foucault (2005) analyzes that:

In disciplinary institutions, the rule of functional locations gradually codifies a space that architecture generally left free and ready for various uses. Certain places are defined to satisfy not only the need to monitor, to break up dangerous communications, but also to create a useful space (FOUCAULT, 2005, p. 123).

In order to exercise total disciplinary control, Foucault (2005) cites the correct use of time, with rigid schedules that are always repetitive and constant. This is why the timetable is a perfect mechanism for disciplinary control.

It is in the control of time and space, carried out by disciplinary procedures, that disciplinary power takes place. In the disciplinary condition, the body subjected to surveillance and control techniques tends to become a docile body. In the procedures reported by Foucault on torture, these practices tore bodies apart. But in disciplinary practices, bodies are given the purpose of guaranteeing maximum results for those who appropriate disciplinary powers.

4.4. Resistance as self-care and practice

According to Wanzeler (2011), the formula of "occupying oneself with oneself", that is, the *heautou epimeleisthai,* was widely used, according to Foucault, in the so-called Socratic dialogues, which became known mainly with the work of Plato[15] .

---

15 According to Foucault, among the cynics, it was useless to focus on certain natural phenomena, such as the origin of earthquakes, what causes storms, the reasons for the birth of twins. Rather, "we should look at immediate things that concern ourselves and at certain rules by which we can conduct ourselves and control what we do". Foucault dealt with this theme in relation to the Epicureans in his lecture on February 10, 1982. This notion of self-care also appears among the Stoics. Seneca and the

Wanzeler (2011) points out that Foucault's (2006) concern in his task of unveiling the history of the thought of self-care lies in being able to "define the conditions in which human beings problematize what they are, what they do and the world in which they live". In this regard, Foucault (2006) deals with the so-called "rational and voluntary practices by which men not only determine for themselves rules of conduct, but also seek to transform themselves, modify themselves in their singular being, and make of their lives a work that carries certain aesthetic values and corresponds to certain criteria of style" (FOUCAULT, 2006, pp.198199 apud WANZELER, 2011).

Delving deeper into Foucault's (1985) thinking, we feel the need to address an issue that is very relevant to the questions considered by the author.

Concern is directed, above all, at the point where agitations and disturbances occur, bearing in mind the fact that the soul must be corrected if it is to maintain complete control over itself. It is to this point of contact, as the individual's point of weakness, that the attention paid to physical ailments, discomforts and sufferings is directed. The body that the adult has to deal with when he takes care of himself is no longer the young body that used to be trained through gymnastics; it is a fragile, threatened body, riddled with small miseries and which, in turn, threatens the soul less through its overly vigorous demands than through its own weaknesses. (FOUCAULT, 1985, p.62).

According to Wanzeler (2011), the movement to displace the precept of the self must be present at all stages of life, and the very meaning of old age is observed by Foucault as a new type of privilege. Foucault (1985) cites the liberation experienced by old age in relation to physical desires, political and individual ambitions and the acquisition of experience. This concept will greatly contribute to our reflection on resistance as self-care and practice (WANZELER, 2011, p. 59).

By contextualizing in this research the issues related to aging and Foucault's (1985) ideas about the origin of self-care, we propose the following question. Who is today's elderly individual?

When we reflect on the elderly in contemporary times, they are surrounded by subjectivation. Being old in contemporary times means responding to or denying certain practices. Therefore, when we investigate the social representation of the

---

cura sui. Foucault also deals with self-care in "History of Sexuality" III (WANZELER, 2011, p. 29).

elderly in contemporary times, we observe that the elderly express the stimuli, acts and memories that they often don't recognize as their own, but rather accept them in a process of introspection, and then begin to assume the behaviors and responses imposed by the new social order of old age.

We therefore understand that the new construction of the elderly in contemporary times is related to an enunciation. According to Foucault (2008) "an utterance is always an event that neither language nor meaning can exhaust entirely" (FOUCAULT, 2008, p. 32).

Foucault's (2008) discourse reminds us of the possibility that the new construction of the elderly subject is based on statements advocated by the media or ideologies that may be associated with consumption and new technologies or practices that will restore health, youth and eternal life.

The concept of enunciation so well defined by Foucault (2008) could impose a new practice on care, which is characterized by a process of objectification that is produced through innovations in these behaviors, elaborated from methods and products so well idealized by the economic order, in order to build a social representation of the elderly updated with other practices in self-care.

The new elderly person idealized by the media and the new forms of care is the one who frequents leisure spaces, trips, courses and universities. They want to be on social networks and up to date with the new proposals for coexistence between young and old. But let's turn to the long-lived, whose care practices need the help of others, because finitude may be much closer. We're talking about old people whose bodies and memories have already been taken over by the degenerative process and chronic, incapacitating illnesses. What would be the possibility for these shipwrecked people, forgotten by the society that advocates the urgency of eternal life?

Let's take as an element of resistance to self-care, the social memory of old individuals forgotten by society in search of long-lasting aging that pursues the myth of aging reduced to bodies without the marks of time in order to be accepted and meet the dictates of the concept of active aging.

In order for self-care among institutionalized old people who have been forgotten by the new social order of successful old age to be fulfilled, it will be necessary to revisit the theories of Foucault (2005).

For Foucault (2005), power is exercised; it is not the attribute of a specific group, "the individual is an effect of power and, at the same time, insofar as it is an effect of power, it is its intermediary: power passes through the individual it constitutes" (FOUCAULT, 2005, p. 32). In the case of the long-lived and forgotten, they are traversed by this power, taking on the proposed practices or resisting them through their reminiscences.

4.5. Reminiscence and social memory in old age

"In remembrance we find ourselves and our identity" (BOBBIO, 1997, p.55).

Based on Bobbio's thinking (1997), we want to delve into the memories that lead all old people to reconstruct their past and give new meaning to their present.

According to Bosi:

There is a moment when the mature man ceases to be an active member of society, ceases to be a driving force in the present life of his group: in this moment of social old age, however, he has one function left: that of remembering. That of being the memory of the family, of the group, of the institution, of society (BOSI, 1994, p. 63).

In order to delve deeper into the paths that lead us to reflect on the concepts of social memory, it is worth turning to Pollak's (1992) thoughts on aspects related to the construction of memory and social identity.

Pollak (1992) then asks the following questions about the construction of social memory: What, then, are the constitutive elements of memory, individual or collective? Firstly, they are the events we have personally experienced. Secondly, they are the events that I would call "lived by table", in other words, events lived by the group or collectivity to which the person feels they belong (POLLAK, 1992, p. 2).

For Pollak (1992), events in which people don't always take part as protagonists, but which in the imagination develop some affective link to the event itself, make it almost impossible to know whether that person took part or not.

Following Pollak's theories (1992), he comments that "it is perfectly possible that, through political socialization or historical socialization, a phenomenon of projection or identification with a certain past occurs, so strong that we can speak of an almost inherited memory" (POLLAK, 1992, p. 2).

For Bosi (2003), the memory of old people can be seen as a mediator between our generation and the witnesses of the past. It is the informal intermediary of culture, since there are formalized mediators constituted by institutions (the school, the church, the political party, etc.) and there is the transmission of values, contents, attitudes, in short, the constituents of culture.

The author also deals with places of memory, which are memories that are not necessarily linked to the chronological facts of the individual's life. These are facts related to, for example, a childhood vacation spot. Facts that come to mind, regardless of the actual date on which the experience took place (BOSI, 2003).

At a certain point in their lives, but precisely when they reach old age, we see that old people start to resort to memories of the past as if they were better than memories of the present. Considering Pollak's (1992) ideas about what he called "places of memory", it's quite understandable that "places of memory" awaken in the old individual a sense of pleasure and fulfillment of the soul because of events that marked their existence. These reminiscences somehow provide the individual with possibilities to resist the hardships of the degenerative aging process.

In his historical studies, the author also defines that memory undergoes fluctuations that are a function of the moment in which it is articulated, in which it is being expressed. The concerns of the moment constitute an element in the structuring of memory.

Having discussed the concept of social memory, we understand that facts of an individual or collective nature can have an impact on the social construction of memory. Pollak (1992) refers to memory as a constructed phenomenon, since the ways in which it is constructed can be either conscious or unconscious. For the author, what individual memory records, represses, excludes and remembers is obviously the result of real organizational work.

If we relate the ageing process to the phenomenon constructed by the author from the point of view of the conscious or unconscious, we can highlight some mechanisms of resistance that can be developed by old individuals in order to cope with maintaining their state of existence.

Still considering Pollak (1992), he also deals in his research with the meaning of self-image, for him, it is the image that a person acquires throughout their life regarding themselves, the image that they construct and present to others and to themselves, in order to believe in their own representation, but also to be perceived in the way they want by others.

In the aspect related to the image described by the author, we realize that the aging process brings a deterioration of this physical image of subjects aged by time, however, it is necessary to elaborate on the structure of the image and the Self defined in the old subject.

For the construction of identity, the author uses social psychology and partly psychoanalysis. He conceptualizes three essential elements: physical unity - the feeling of physical boundaries, in the case of a person's body, or boundaries of belonging to a group, in the case of a collective; continuity over time, in the physical sense of the word, but also in the moral and psychological sense; and finally, there is the sense of coherence, i.e. that the different elements that make up an individual are effectively unified (POLLAK, 1992, p. 5).

The author then defines memory as a constituent element of the feeling of identity.

Pollak (1992) also emphasizes in his research that when memory and identity are sufficiently constituted, sufficiently instituted, sufficiently tied down, questions from groups outside the organization, problems posed by others, do not provoke the need to rearrange, neither at the level of collective identity nor at the level of individual identity.

Considering all the issues that have led us to reflect on the process of reminiscence and social memory in old age, as well as one of the aspects present in our research that leads us to contextualize the forms of enclosure and the possible aspects of resistance in the shelters of old people, these questions may allow us to build an ethic of existence in institutionalized old age.

4.6. Enclosure x Reminiscence and Resistance: An Ethic of Existence

> The doors of the asylum, the walls of the prison disappeared, giving way to free conversations in which Greeks and Romans discussed the best ways to lead their lives (...). The landscape of confinement gives way to the luminous freedom of the subject (EWALD, 1984).

It is interesting to note that in the various conferences, theses and reflections developed by Foucault on power, enclosure and resistance, he leads us to think about questions that we have not yet found answers to.

Fischer (1999) asks how the insane come to be considered "mentally ill"? In order to identify the discourse, Foucault (1997), in 'The History of Madness', analyzes medical discourses and internment practices, considering the social instances involved - churches, family, medicine, justice - from the Renaissance to the beginning of the 19th century.

The creation of the first hospitals, in the 17th century, instituted social exclusion, based mainly on moral criteria: the inmates were prostitutes (and all those who acquired venereal diseases), deviants, sexual perverts, sorcerers and magicians, libertines and, finally, the insane, until then not seen as mentally ill (FISCHER, 1999, p. 45).

Foucault analyzes that in the 18th century, however, medical discourse distinguished madness from other types of "moral errors", classifying it as a product of man's relationship with his environment and identifying it as a phenomenon that takes place within the subject himself (FISCHER, 1999, p. 45).

Considering this last analysis by Foucault, described by Fischer (1999), let's explore the institutions for the elderly and confinement measures. In order to support this analysis, it is considered necessary to appropriate the reflections of the history of the creation of institutions of confinement, in order to justify the enclosure of frail old people. Measures of confinement and enclosure used these methods to hide decrepitude and the ills of old age.

Frederic Gros (2004) comments that if Foucault wrote a "History of Madness", it was not to make a history of psychiatry; if he wrote "Words and Things", it was not to make a history of the human sciences; if he studied the Greeks and Romans, it was not to make a history of Hellenistic and Latin philosophy, his reflections, his words are a philosophical, ethical and political position: Foucault invents a philosophy that liberates our own existence from ourselves or from the prison of our "subjectivity", which, socially and historically constructed, is nevertheless experienced as a natural and universal substance (GROS, 2004 apud SOUZA FILHO, 2007).

When discussing power, enclosure, resistance and freedom, Foucault (2010) is emphatic in stating that power is productive, power manufactures, because if power only had the function of repressing, if power only used censorship, exclusion, impediment, repression, it would be weak. If power is strong, it is because it produces effects of resistance, freedom and desire.

In Histoire de la sexualite: la volonte de savoir, Foucault states that the forces of resistance are based precisely on the point where power invests, namely life and man as a living being (FOUCAULT, 2010, p. 158).

Contextualizing power and resistance, Souza Filho (2007) asks the following question: Is it possible to constitute the subject without subjection?

The author explains that for Foucault (2004) this implies the transformation of the subject as the object of knowledge, the object of their own truth, with freedom being built in a process, in a life constructed in the way each one determines.

This is what I have tried to reconstruct: the formation and development of a practice of the self which aims to constitute oneself as the artisan of the beauty of one's own life (FOUCAULT, 2004. p. 244).

In "Surveillance and Punishment", Foucault (2005) discusses how prison measures turn man into an object, defining it as "the political history of bodies".

For Fischer (1999), in his history of the microphysics of punitive power in "Surveillance and Punishment", Foucault describes the foundations of the modern "soul" that constitutes us in contemporary times, as described in the following excerpt:

(...) the man they tell us about and invite us to liberate is already in himself the effect of a subjection much deeper than himself. A 'soul' inhabits him and brings him into existence, which is itself a grip on the domination exercised by power over the body. The soul, effect and instrument of a political anatomy; the soul, prison of the body. (FOUCAULT, 1987, pp.31-32)

Enclosure, resistance and reminiscence alone are no longer enough for the old bodies in asylums.

Souza Filho (2007) deals with self-care in his article, posing the following question. "And because self-care as a practice of freedom is an ethical problem - how to act? This is the question of the ethical subject - self-care requires techniques. The author reports that Foucault deals with some of them in his enchanting reading of the "life manuals" of antiquity: reading, writing, dream interpretation, meditation, reflection, care of the body (sleep, physical exercise, food, drink, excretion, sexual relations, etc.). They are all techniques for constituting the self as an object of radical action: an object of subjectivation-other. Techniques of working on oneself as a place of experience, of rehearsals of existence.

4.7. Movie Exterminating Angel - scene three (the resistance)

Finally, we analyze scene three of the film "The Exterminating Angel". The final scene portrays the repercussions of the process of confinement and the consequences that this process has on the human condition. In this scene, the characters go through several days of confinement and, as a result, they begin a process of loss and temporal disorientation. Episodes of illness, hysteria, psychic and emotional imbalance take over the scene.

The characters go from introspection to existential chaos, in the face of discomfort, conflict, confusion, disorder, suffocation and anguish. Different ways of externalizing the pulses of life and death are expressed, from the demonstration of beliefs, faith and superstitions, through religious rites, to the catharsis that emerged through verbal insults, physical attacks, betrayals, addictions and delirium. The loss of freedom in Bunuel's film illustrates the crises of self-care that can occur when subjects are captured and remain in stages of confinement.

According to Schaefer and Farias (2014), imprisonment is a singular and radical experience, pushing the subject to their limits as they are confronted with a situation from which they cannot leave of their own volition. This sudden change of life is felt as violence.

In these spaces of imprisonment, individuals seem to be watched and, why not say it, controlled in their actions and emotions. Schaefer and Farias (2014) also suggest that imprisonment, in addition to depriving people of the freedom to come and go, also deprives them of other elementary functions such as thought, i.e. thought can collapse.

But how can the imposition of disciplinary power in nursing homes be resisted?

In "The Ethics of Self-Care as a Practice of Freedom" - an interview with Foucault on January 20, 1984 - the notion of resistance is explicitly taken up and reworked. The notion of resistance accompanies this theoretical shift in the axis of power. When Foucault (1988) is asked about "a certain deficiency" in his problematics, more specifically, in relation to a "conception of resistance to power", he says: "this brings me back to the problem of what I understand by power" (FOUCAULT, 1988, pp. 11-12 apud BAMPI, 2002).

Returning to the scene of resistance in Bunuel's film, all the characters, faced with confinement, are trying to find a consensual way out to reverse the chaos and the different expressions of emotions, which are laid bare when the masks, wrappings and disguises that cover social roles crumble, and individualism, selfishness, cruelty, vanity and pride emerge.

At one point, while everyone seems to be regaining their sanity and emotional balance, an attempt is made to go back in time to the dinner offered by the hosts. It is at this point that the tensions give way to rationality. The images start to become clearer, reminiscences seem to emerge.

The house opens up, and all the residents and guests seem to harmonize in the hope of better days.

5. FINAL CONSIDERATIONS

This Master's thesis, entitled ***Institutionalization of the elderly: A space of reminiscence and resistance?*** It is a proposal to better investigate the spaces where old people are sheltered, where the conformities of frail subjects, taken over by the process of degenerative ageing, are combined with the wait for finitude; facts that portray in reality the consequences of a stigmatized ageing that is fraught with situations involving the sublimation of desires, apathy to the facts of everyday life, submission to imposed orders and neglect of the rights won in the democratic processes that the country has gone through since the promulgation of the 1988 Federal Constitution.

Having made a theoretical, reflective and critical study of the asylum model in old age, we have identified that institutions for the elderly still retain in themselves and in their culture historical aspects dating back to the 19th century. These institutions are still preceded by rigid rules and discipline that are no longer appropriate today. Disciplinary and behavioral procedures are still part of the institutions of old, a theme that has been subjected to an interdisciplinary conceptual analysis in the area of psychoanalysis and society.

The study achieved its objectives by situating socio-historical aspects as a means of contextualizing the formation of institutions for the care of the elderly in Brazil and demonstrating how practices based on institutionalization are perpetuated and how public policies, although making progress, do not problematize the effects of this process on subjects and subjectivities. This problem is relevant because it will be exacerbated by an ageing population and a falling birth rate in the country. Specifically, the study tried to describe gerontological practices in ILPIs, according to official policy documents instituted in Brazil; it also discussed questions about the discomfort of growing old in contemporary times and analyzed the effects of confinement and the possible ways of resisting and sustaining reminiscences and social memories.

The theoretical basis followed concepts of total institution and degradation of the self, according to Goffman's analysis, concepts of power, disciplinary power and biopower, in Foucault's view, and the concepts of malaise in culture, the pulse of life and the pulse of death from Freud's perspective and contemporary psychoanalytic authors. Methodologically, these conceptual tools were able to bring together critical perspectives on the subject of the old people's home, through the use of surrealist cinema as a means of illustrating and metaphorizing the proposed theme.

The study articulated reflections on total institutions and disciplinary practices, pointing to the degradation of the Self and the docilization of bodies, linked to strategies of biopower and biopolitics, in such a way that aging is forbidden and rejuvenation appears as a maxim to be followed. Aging and dying are postponed in favor of active aging that supports consumerism and avoids decrepitude, a fragile aging, an old age that is reserved for nursing homes, when there is helplessness or when families delegate the care of their elderly to charitable or private entities.

Shelters for the elderly are characterized by a microstructure of institutionalized power where docile bodies must submit to obedience in order to guarantee their survival. Constructing an analytical and critical position on the asylum space, linked to the power of domination over fragile individuals, sought to promote the revision of a conceptualization of the place of the elderly in contemporary society.

Considering the historical aspects described in the research on the emergence of asylums, we highlight Goffman's thinking. According to the author, in total institutions the individual perceives himself as institutionalized, having to give up comforts and habits. They take on the impact of the new social dimension established by institutionalization and its disciplinary rules. In a nursing home, the elderly person feels like they are in an oppressive space, since the inmates are forced to work together and are supervised by one or more people, remaining under surveillance as a means of ensuring what has been indicated and demanded.

In Goffman's theoretical reflection, he highlights the mortification of the self in confinement spaces, when the subject ceases to be someone and becomes part of something, in other words, their "self" gives way to the goals of the institution, giving way to the process of institutionalization. There is a power that is expressed in a condition of

a repressive and mutilating power of the self. In these closed institutions, there is a progressive change in individuals' respect for themselves and for others.

Goffman provided support for our research into the aspects surrounding the historical construction of old people's homes in Brazil, characterizing the dilemmas produced by the issues of order and social interaction that are kept under control.

In Foucault, we seek to understand the power that is established in these closed spaces, understanding the notion of power as a bundle of relationships that constitute a system of control networks over individuals subjugated to disciplinary rules. Institutional spaces are seen as small, hierarchical micro-powers where domination over bodies is structured on the basis of the institutionalization of rules, docilizing bodies that become malleable to the instituted practices.

As Foucault says, disciplinary institutions are not limited to confinement alone, but rather to a genealogy of punitive power for those individuals who do not want to reproduce disciplinary behaviors, nor do they want to execute the rules that have been instituted. In this context, control is established through fear and submission, which is more violent than confinement itself.

The idea of supplication, as described by Foucault and practiced in the 18th century, has given way to the punishment of the soul, psychological punishment with the use of science and politics in contemporary times, applying the power of coercion on weak individuals to docile bodies.

Based on the author's analysis, we believe that power uses the classification of individuals in order to better control the bodies produced by a sequentialist society, where active old people stay in public spaces or in their homes enjoying the benefits produced by the consumer system, while frail and sick old people are separated and taken to confinement institutions.

The social, economic and political system depends on a construction to effectively exert domination over people. This system develops mechanisms of control, mechanisms of power and mechanisms of domination in order to better control its own species, selecting those who will be able to age well socially and those who will have to live an excluded old age.

The concepts of biopower and biopolitics, so well defined by Foucault, have helped us to reflect on how politics can exercise control over the lives of individuals, populations, peoples and nations, through rules of domination and control over bodies, often with subtle and almost imperceptible resources of submission.

There is an aestheticization of everyday life in contemporary times that is crossed by values of success, beauty, the perfect body, happiness and rejuvenation products to be consumed, which perpetuate a feeling that the subject cannot get old. This malaise associated with ageing is perpetuated by a media culture, a world that produces individualistic, narcissistic and unsympathetic beings who are averse to ageing and see old age as something undesirable.

When we reflect on the elderly in nursing homes, we see that the malaise is expressed not only in an institutionalized old age, but above all in a decrepit old age, crossed by suffering, by the being that does not reinvigorate itself and which in common sense is associated with despair, loneliness and the sadness of growing old. This malaise is even more insidious in the institutionalized elderly, who remain oblivious to themselves and their surroundings, except through mechanisms of resistance and reminiscences that preserve them as desiring subjects.

Therefore, in the spaces of the ILPIs, it is necessary to increase and elaborate the planning of group techniques that direct the institutionalized elderly individuals to the construction of their affective memories, memories that rescue family relationships, as well as facts arising from reminiscences that are relevant to the life contexts of the aging subjects.

Nursing homes need to establish a constant dialogue with society in order to keep alive the pulse of life of the elderly living in long-term care facilities.

We must analyze nursing homes as a space of great importance for caring for the elderly, who deserve a comprehensive care process with qualified professionals who are sensitive to the aging process, resources that will help nursing home residents maintain their functionality and potential.

When we turn to Freud's impulses, we realize that the author gives a very consistent treatment to the theory of impulses. Through the concept of pulse, Freud problematizes the question of a life and death force, the impetus that falls on the individual as an impact and that instigates them and leads them towards some action.

For Freud, unlike instincts, drive is a constant force. The drive is not a variable force; on the contrary, it is a constant force that can push in a constructive or destructive direction. Every human being is seized by something that instigates them at all times. The drive demands specific work from individuals, which takes place through symptoms, when the subject cannot find the means to express their desires or their way of being or feeling, or through sexuality and investment in life, pleasure and the affections that organize existence.

For Freud, sexuality is a drive sexuality. It is a sexuality that constantly challenges individuals, characterizing the drive and the object of desire, and then establishing the relationship with what manifests itself as the object that causes desire and mobilizes living.

Considering Freud's pulse theory, what is fundamental about each pulse is the back and forth in which it is structured. A back and forth that mobilizes the life and living of beings in relationship with themselves and with others.

Answering the initial research question, which asks ***Institutionalization of old people: A space for reminiscence and resistance? It*** is necessary to create a view of aging in which there is room for decrepitude, for an expected degeneration of bodies in late aging, which can be welcomed and cared for in a context of integrality and intergenerationality. Ageing must be a continuous process of life, with subjective and social facts and acts that make us the protagonists of the social construction of old age, something that can only happen through an "ethic of existence", through care that gives space to desire, to resist and to remember.

REFERENCES

ARIES, Philippe. **Historia Social da Crianga e da Famflia**. 2 ed. Rio de Janeiro: LTC, 1981.

AUMONT, J.; BERGALA, A.; MARIE, M.; VERNET, M (1994). **The aesthetics of film**. Campinas - SP: Papirus, 2011.

AUMONT, J.; MARIE, M. **A analise do filme.** Lisbon: Texto e Grafia, 2009.

BAMPI, Lisete. **Government, subjectivation and resistance in Foucault.** In: Education and Reality. Jan/Jun 2003, 27(1): 127-150. Available at: seer.ufrgs.br /index.php/educacaoerealidade/article/view/25941/15204, Accessed on July 15, 2018.

BAUDIN, Talita. **Old age and institutionalization**: **scenes from life in a shelter** / Talita Baldin. - 2016. 123 f. Supervisor: Paulo Eduardo Viana Vidal. Dissertation (Master's) - Universidade Federal Fluminense, Instituto de Ciencias Humanas e Filosofia, Departamento de Psicologia, 2016. Master's thesis 123f.

BEAUVOIR, SIMONE de (1970). **Old Age**. Rio de Janeiro: Nova Fronteira, 1990.

BILLOUET, Pierre. **Foucault.** Sao Paulo: Estagao Liberdade, 2003.

BIRMAN, Joel. **Malaise today: psychoanalysis and the new forms of subjectivation.** 3. ed. Rio de Janeiro: Civilizagao Brasileira, 2001. Available at: http://pepsic.bvsalud.org/pdf/psyche/v11n20/v11n20a13.pdf. Accessed on July 12, 2018.

BOBBIO, Noberto. **The Time of Memory.** Rio de Janeiro: Campus, 1997.

BORGES, M. B. O. **The production of knowledge on human ageing**: historical and social aspects. Faculty of Health Sciences, Psychology course. Monograph 2007.

BOSCHETTI, Ivanete. **Social security in Brazil: achievements and limits to its realization.** In: CFESS. Social Work: Social Rights and Professional Competences. Brasilia, CFESS and ABEPSS, 2010.

BOSI, Eclea. **Memoria e Sociedade:** Lembranga de Velhos . 2. ed., Sao Paulo: T.A. Queiroz, 1994.

BOSI, Eclea. **O tempo vivo da memória:** ensaios de psicologia social. Sao Paulo: Atelie, 2003.

BRASIL. **Brasil 2050 [recurso eletronico]: desafios de uma nagao que envelhece** / Chamber of Deputies, Center for Strategic Studies and Debates, Legislative Consultancy; rapporteur Cristiane Brasil; legislative consultants Alexandre Candido de Souza (coord.), Alberto Pinheiro ... [et al.]. - Brasilia: Camara dos Deputados, Edigoes Camara, 2017. - (Strategic studies series; n. 8 PDF). Available at: www2.camara.leg.br/a-camara/estruturaadm/altosestudos/pdf/brasil- 2050-os./view. Accessed on June 3, 2018.

BRAZIL. **Constitution of the Federative Republic of Brazil.** Diario Oficial da Uniao, Section 1, p. 1, October 5, 1988. Available at <http://www.lexml.gov.br/urn/urn:lex:br:federal:constituicao:1988-10-05;1988>. Accessed on June 3, 2018.

BRAZIL. **DECREE No. 1.948, of July 3, 1996**. Available at HTTP://www.aposfurnas.org.br/?q=node/190. Accessed June 15, 2017.

BRAZIL. Brazilian Institute of Geography and Statistics (IBGE). **National Household Sample Survey.** Summary of Social Indicators. Ministry of Planning, Organization and Management. Demographic and socio-economic information, 2011.

BRAZIL. Brazilian Institute of Geography and Statistics (IBGE). **An analysis of the living conditions of the Brazilian population**. Summary of Social Indicators. Ministry of Planning, Organization and Management. Demographic and socio-economic information. Studies and Research Series, demographic and socio-economic information, No. 29, 2012. Available at: https://biblioteca.ibge.gov.br/ visualizacao/livros/liv62715.pdf. Accessed on June 3, 2018.

BRAZIL. **Law n. 8.842, of January 4, 1994.** Provides for the national policy for the elderly, creates the National Council for the Elderly and makes other provisions. **Diario Oficial da Uniao**, Section 1, p. 77, January 5, 1994. Available at <http://www.lexml. gov.br/urn/urn:lex:br:federal:lei:1994-01-04;8842>. Accessed on April 15, 2018.

BRAZIL. **Law No. 10.741, of October 1, 2003.** Diario Oficial da Uniao, Section 1, p.1, October 3, 2003. Available at <http://www.planalto.gov.br/ccivil_03/leis/ 2003/L10.741.htm>. Accessed on June 3, 2018.

BRAZIL. Ministry of Health. National Health Surveillance Agency (Anvisa). **Collegiate Board Resolution No. 283, of September 26, 2005**. Approves the technical regulation that defines operating standards for long-stay institutions for the elderly. Diario Oficial da Uniao, Brasilia, September 27, 2005. Available at: <www.portalsaude.gov.br>. Accessed on June 3, 2018.

BRAZIL. Ministry of Social Development. **Ordinance No. 2.854, of July 20, 2000.** Diario Oficial da Uniao July 21, 2000. [Accessed on July 3, 2010]. Available at <http://www.renipac.org.br/port2854.html>. Accessed on June 3, 2018.

BRAZIL. Ministry of Social Development. **Ordinance No. 2.874, of August 30, 2000. Amends Ordinance No. 2.854, of July 20, 2000.** Available at <https://www.mds.gov.br/webarquivos/legislacao/assistencia_social/portarias/2000/Portaria%20no%202.874-%20de%2030%20de%20agosto%20de%202000.pdf>. Accessed on June 5, 2018.

BRAZIL. Secretariat for Social Assistance Policies. Social Assistance Policy Development Department, Elderly Care Management. Ordinance No. 73 of May 10, 2001. **Norms for the Operation of Services for the Elderly in Brazil**. Available at: <http://www.saudeidoso. icict.fiocruz.br/index.php?pag=polit>. Accessed on June 3, 2018.

BRIGIDO, Edimar Inocencio. **Michel Foucault**: an analysis of power. In: Rev. Direito Econ. Socioambiental, Curitiba, v. 4 . n. 1. pp. 56-75,, jan./jun. 2013. Available at: http://www.egov.ufsc.br/portal/sites/default/files/direitoeconomico- 12702.pdf . Accessed on July 11, 2018.

BUNEL, L. **Biography.** Available at: <https://pt.wikipedia.org/wiki/Luis_Bu%C3% B1uel>. Accessed on June 3, 2018.

CAMARANO, A. A. **Aging of the Brazilian population: a demographic contribution.** Textos para Discussao no 858. Rio de Janeiro: IPEA, Jan. 2012. Available at <http://repositorio.ipea.gov.br/bitstream/11058/2091/1/TD_858.pdf>. Accessed on: March 25, 2018. Accessed on April 20, 2018.

CAMPOS, Erico B. V. **On the actuality of malaise**. In: Psyche - Ano XI- n° 20 - Sao Paulo - jan-jun/2007 - pp. 185-189. Available at: http://pepsic.bvsalud.org/pdf/psyche/v11n20/v11n20a13.pdf. Accessed on April 20, 2018.

CANDIDO, INA. **Plato's Cave and the cinema**. In: Blog Sagaz. Unraveling society and its culture, May 14, 2011. Available at: <https://sagaz.wordpress.com/2011/05/14/a-caverna-de-platao-e-o-cinema/>. Accessed on June 3, 2018.

CARVALHO, Antonio. **Social Assistance Policy for the Elderly.** Master's dissertation, Public Policies and Local Development Program, Escola Superior de Ciencias da Santa Casa de Misericordia de Vitoria - EESCAM. Supervisor: Prof. Dr. Alacir Ramos Silva. Vitoria, 2011. Available at: http://www.emescam.br/arquivos/pos/stricto/dissertacoes/56_Antonio_Carvalho.pdf , accessed June 17, 2018.

CASTILHO. G. M. **Psicanalise e Velhice.** Federal University of Rio de Janeiro, Center for Human Sciences and Philosophy. Institute of Ps1d:1 Logia Postgraduate Program in Psychoanalytic Theory. Doctoral thesis 2011. Available at: http://pantheon.ufrj.br/bitstream/11422/3776/3/775428.pdf. Accessed on June 3, 2018.

DANNER, Fernando. **The Meaning of Biopolitics in Michel Foucault**. Revista Estudos Filosoficos n° 4 /2010, pp. 143 - 157. Available at: https://www.ufsj.edu.br/portal2-repositorio/File/revistaestudosfilosoficos/art9-rev4.pdf Accessed on June 03, 2018.

DEBERT, G. G. (Org.) **Anthropology and old age.** Campinas: IFCH/UNICAMP, 1998. (Textos Didaticos).
. **The invention of old age and the rearticulation of forms of consumption and political demands.** In: Cadernos Pagu (21), 2003. Available at: http://www.scielo.br/pdf/%0D/cpa/n21/n21a07.pdf . Accessed on May 10, 2018.

EWALD, Frangois. **Michel Foucault** . In: ESCOBAR, Carlos Henrique de. (Org.)

Michel Foucault: The dossier - last interviews . Rio de Janeiro: Taurus, 1984.

FEATHERSTONE, M. **Consumer culture and postmodernism.** Sao Paulo: Studio Nobel, 1995.

FELIPE. T.W.S. e SOUSA. S.M.N. **A construgao da categoria velhice e seus significados.** Revista eletronica de humanidades do curso de Ciencias Sociais. UNIFAP-Macapa, v7, n2, p.19-33, July, December, 2014.

FILHO, Alipio de Sousa. **Foucault: self-care and freedom, or freedom and an agomstic.** (Paper presented at the IV Michel Foucault International Colloquium. April 2007, Natal - RN) Available at: http://www.redehumanizasus.net/sites/ default/files/foucault20o20cuidado20de20si20e20a20liberdade.pdf. Accessed on March 27, 2015.

FILIZZOLA, Mario. **Old age in Brazil:** ageism and civilization. Rio de Janeiro: cia Brasileira de Artes e Cultura, 1972. 485p.

FISCHER, Rosa Maria Bueno. **Foucault and the desirable knowledge of the subject.** Educagao & Realidade - v.1, n.1 (feb. 1976). Porto Alegre: Educagao & Realidade Porto Alegre v.24 n.1 p.5-183 jan.ljun. 1999. Available: www.seer.ufrgs.br/ educacaoerealidade/issue/download/2584/369 .Accessed on July 09, 2018.

FOUCAULT, Michel. **The archaeology of knowledge.** Trad. Luiz Felipe Baeta Neves. 7. ed. Rio de Janeiro: Forense Universitaria, 2008.

. **The analytic philosophy of politics**. In: MOTTA, M. B. (org.). Etica, sexualidade, politica. 2 ed., Rio de Janeiro: Forense Universitaria, 2006. pp.198-199.

. (1975). **Surveillance and Punishment: the birth of the prison**. Petropolis: Vozes, 2005. 288p.

_____ . **The Hermeneutics of the Subject**. Sao Paulo: Martins Fontes, 2004. p.616.

. **Microphysics of Power.** Rio de Janeiro: Graal, (1979/2002).

. **Dits et Ecrits II** - 1976-1988. Editions Gallimard, 2001.

. **Words and things:** an archaeology of the human sciences. 8ª Ed. Sao Paulo, Martins Fontes, 1999.

. **The ethic of care of the self as a practice of freedom**. In: BERNAUER, J. and RASMUSSEN, D.(eds). The final Foucault. Cambridge: MIT Press, 1988, pp. 1-20

. **History of Sexuality I: the Will to Know.** Rio de Janeiro: Graal, 1976.

. **Mental Illness and Psychology.** Rio de Janeiro: Editora Tempo Brasileiro, 1962.

FREUD, Sigmund. **Malaise in Civilization** (Brazilian Standard Edition of the Complete Psychological Works of Sigmund Freud, Vol. 21). Rio Janeiro: Imago, 1996/1987 (Originally published in 1930[1929]).

. **La interpretacion de los suenos** (Obras Completas, Vol. 5, pp. 345-670). Buenos Aires, Argentina: Amorrortu, 2007 (Originally published in 1900).

. **Sexuality in the etiology of neurosis**. In: Brazilian Standard Edition of the Complete Works of Sigmund Freud. Rio de Janeiro: Imago, 1898/1976.

. **Terminable and interminable analysis**. In: Brazilian Standard Edition of the Complete Works of Sigmund Freud, vol. XXIII. Rio de Janeiro: Imago, 1937/1975.

Freud's Psychoanalytic Method, Complete Works, 1902[1904]. Available at: http://caece.opac.com.ar/gsdl/collect/apuntes/index/ assoc/HASH011e.dir/doc.pdf. Accessed on June 12, 2018.

. **Studies on Hysteria (1893-1895).** Rio de Janeiro: Imago, 1976. v. XVIII.

. **On Narcissism: an introduction.** In: Complete Works. Direction and translation by Jayme Salomao. v.14. Rio de Janeiro: Imago, 1970[1919],

. **The value of life.** Interview given to journalist George Silvester Viereck in 1926. Translated by Paulo Cezar Souza, on the Blog Semiotica & Pisicanalise. 9Posted in June 2011) Available at: http://semipsica.blogspot.com/2011/07/entrevista-com-freud-1926-o-valor-da.html. Accessed on June 11, 2018.

FREYRE, Gilberto. **Sobrados e Mucambos.** 9 ed. Rio de Janeiro: Record, 1990.

FROEMMING. L.S. **Montage in cinema and free association in psychoanalysis**. Federal University of Rio Grande do Sul. Institute of Psychology. Postgraduate Course in Developmental Psychology. Doctoral thesis, 2002. Available at: http://www.lume.ufrgs.br/handle/10183/2905. Accessed June 10, 2017.

FULGENCIO, Leopoldo. **The speculative method in Freud**, Sao Paulo: Edusp, 2008.

GARCIA-ROZA, Luiz Alfredo. **Lost and found.** Sao Paulo: Companhia das Letras, 2001.

GOFFMAN, Erving. **Asylums, prisons and convents**. Sao Paulo: Perspectiva, 2015/2008/1987.

GOLDFARB, Delia Catullo. **Body, time and ageing.** Master's dissertation, Clinical Psychology Program, PUC-SP, under the supervision of Prof. Dr. Renato Mezan, 1997. Available at: http://www.redpsicogerontologia.net/xxfiles/ Livro%20em%20PDF.pdf. Accessed on July 12, 2018.

GROISMAN, Daniel. **The childhood of the asylum: the institutionalization of old age in Rio de Janeiro at the turn of the century.** Supervisor: Sergio Luis Carrara. Dissertation (master's) Rio de Janeiro - State University of Rio de Janeiro, Institute of Social Medicine, 1999a. 125 f.. Available at: http://bases.bireme.br/cgi-bin/wxislind.exe/iah/online/?IsisScript=iah/iah.xis&src=google&base=LILACS&lang=p &nextAction=lnk&exprSearch=254511&indexSearch=ID. Accessed February 11, 2018.

. **Two approaches to old people's homes:** from the Santa Genoveva clinic to the history of the institutionalization of old age. In: cadernos pagu (13) 1999b : pp. 161-190. Available at: file:///C:/Users/User/Desktop/tudo/Curso%20cuidadores %20de%20idosos%202018/Pagamentos/cadpagu_1999_13_6_GROISMAN.pdf . Accessed July 05, 2018.

GROS, Frederic. **Situation of the course.** In: FOUCAULT, Michel. The Hermeneutics of the Subject. Sao Paulo: Martins Fontes, 2004. p.616.

HADDAD, E. G. M. **A ideologia da velhice.** Sao Paulo: Cortez, 1986.

HATHAWAY, Gisela. **Fundamental rights and guarantees of the elderly in Brazil.** In: Brazil 2050 [electronic resource] : challenges of an ageing nation / Chamber of Deputies, Center for Strategic Studies and Debates, Legislative Consultancy; rapporteur Cristiane Brasil; legislative consultants Alexandre Candido de Souza (coord.), Alberto Pinheiro. [et al.]. - Brasilia : Camara dos Deputados, Edigoes Camara, 2017. - (Serie estudos estrategicos; n. 8 PDF).

KARSCH, U. (org.) **Dependent elderly: families and caregivers.** Cad. Saude Publica, Rio de Janeiro, 19(3):861-866, mai-jun, 2003.

KARSCH, U. (org.), **Aging with Dependence: Revealing Caregivers.** Sao Paulo, EDUC, 1998.

KUCHEMANN, B. A. **Population aging, care and citizenship: old dilemmas and new challenges.** Society and State. Brasilia: v. 27, n. 1 jan-abr. 2012. Available at: <http://www.scielo.br/scielo.php?pid=S0102-69922012000100010& script=sci_arttext>. Accessed June 3, 2018.

KURZ, ROBERT. **The biologization of the social world undergoes a new 'disenchantment'**. Special interview for Folha. Sao Paulo, Sunday, July 7, 1996. Available at: https://www1.folha.uol.com.br/fsp/1996/7/07/ mais!/13.html . Accessed on July 14, 2018.

LACAN, Jacques. **The Seminar: Book V - The Formations of the Unconscious.** Rio de Janeiro: Jorge Zahar, 1999.

LACAN, Jacques. **The Seminar: Book 11: The Four Fundamental Concepts of Psychoanalysis.** Rio de Janeiro: Zahar, 1988 (Seminar given in 1964).

LEMOS, Moises Fernandes. **Psychoanalysis and Cinema: in search of an approximation** / Moises Fernandes Lemos - 2014. 157 f. Supervisor: Prof. Dr. Cristovao Giovani Burgarelli. Thesis (Doctorate) - Federal University of Goias, Faculty of Education, 2014. [manuscript] Available at: https://repositorio.bc.ufg.br/tede/bitstream/ tede/3406/5/Tese%20Moises%20Fernandes%20Lemos%20-%202014.pd. Accessed on April 30, 2018.

LENOIR, Remi. **Sociological Object and Social Problem.** In: MERLLIE, Dominique. Initiation to Sociological Practice. Petropolis: Vozes, 1996. p. 59 - 106.

LIMA, Lais de. **Review of Civilization's Malaise. Word and Listening Blog.**

Sunday, 17/06/2007. Available at: http://www.palavraescuta.com.br/textos/o-mal-estar-na-civilizacao-1930-resenha . Accessed on June 11, 2018.

LIMA, Maria Amelia Ximenes Correia. **Institutionalized doing: the daily life of asylums.** Master's thesis. Sao Paulo (SP): PEPGG / PUC-SP, 2005. Available at: https://tede2.pucsp.br/handle/handle/12403.

LUCCHESI, Geraldo. **Population ageing: prospects for SUS.** In: Brazil 2050 [electronic resource] : challenges of an ageing nation / Chamber of Deputies, Center for Strategic Studies and Debates, Legislative Consultancy; rapporteur Cristiane Brasil; legislative consultants Alexandre Candido de Souza (coord.), Alberto Pinheiro. [et al.]. - Brasilia: Camara dos Deputados, Edigoes Camara, 2017. - (Serie estudos estrategicos; n. 8 PDF).

MAIA, Antonio C. **On Foucault's analysis of power.** Tempo Social. Rev. Sociol. USP, S. Paulo, 7(1-2): 83-103, October 1995.

MESSY, J. **The elderly person does not exist.** Sao Paulo: Aleph, 1993.

MINAYO, M. C. S.; COIMBRA, jr. **Between freedom and dependence: reflections on the social phenomenon of ageing.** In: MINAYO, M. C. S.; COIMBRA JR., C. E. A (Orgs.) Anthropology, health and ageing (pp. 11-24). Rio de Janeiro: Editora FIOCRUZ, 2002.

MIRANDA, Heraldo de Cristo. **Foucault and Goffman: on institutions and powers.** In Sapere aude magazine - Belo Horizonte, v. 8, n. 16, p. 381-394, Aug./Dec. 2017 . Available at: periodicos.pucminas.br/index.php/SapereAude/article/.../ P...2017v8n16p381/12757 . Accessed on July 11, 2018.

MONNERAT, Giselle Lavinas; SOUZA, Rosimary Gongalves. **From Social Security to intersectorality: reflections on the integration of social policies in Brazil**. In: Rev. katalysis, vol.14 no.1 Florianopolis Jan./June 2011. Available at: http://www.scielo. br/scielo.php?script=sci_arttext&pid=S1414-49802011000100005 . Accessed on September 3, 2017.

MOREIRA, Viginia; NOGUEIRA; Fernanda Nicia Nunes. **From the undesirable to the inevitable: the lived experience of the stigma of growing old in contemporary times.** In: Psicol. USP vol.19 no.1 Sao Paulo Jan./Mar. 2008. Available at: http://www.scielo.br/scielo.php?script=sci_arttext&pid=S0103-65642008000100009. Accessed on July 12, 2018.

OLIVEIRA, Andre Renato de. **Thought based on the mechanism of the unconscious in the first Freudian topic**. Master's dissertation State University of Campinas, Institute of Philosophy and Human Sciences. Campinas, SP: [s.n], 2015.

WHO. **World Report on Ageing and Health.** 2015. Available at: http://sbgg.org.br/wp-content/uploads/2015/10/OMS-ENVELHECIMENTO-2015-port.pdf . Accessed on May 19, 2017.

UN. **World Population Prospects: The 2017 Revision.** Available at:

https://esa.un.org/unpd/wpp/Publications/Files/WPP2017_KeyFindings.pdf. Accessed on September 5, 2017.

POLLAK, Michael. **Historical Studies.** Rio de Janeiro, vol. 5, n. 10, 1992, p. 200212. Available at: http://www.pgedf.ufpr.br/memoria%20e%20identidadesocial%20A%20capraro%202.pdf. Accessed on July 9, 2018.

PRIORI, Mary Del. **Conversations on the history of the body.** In: Corpo para que te quero? Uses, abuses and disuses. VILHENA, Junia de; NOVAES, Joana de Vilhena. Rio de Janeiro: Editora Appris/Editora PUC Rio, 2012, v. 1, pp. 239-248.

SANTOS. Claudia Rodrigues de Souza dos. **The elderly in Brazil: from unequipped old age to old age with rights?** Course Conclusion Paper for the Latu Sensu Postgraduate Course in Family Therapy at the Candido Mendes University. Supervisor Prof. Diva Nereida M. Maranhao. Rio de Janeiro, 2007. Available at: http://www.avm.edu.br/monopdf/3/claudia%20rodrigues%20de%20souza%20dos%20santos.pdf January/2007, accessed June 17, 2018.

SANTOS. S. S.; CARLOS. S. A. **Clinical observations on the value of reminiscences in the aging process**. Barbaroi no.35 Santa Cruz do Sul dec. 2011.

SCHAEFER, Patricia. FARIAS, Francisco Ramos. **The experience of imprisonment from the perspective of the tragic and the baroque.** In: Psicanalise & Barroco em revista v.12, n. 1: 13-31, jul. 2014. Available at: www.seer.unirio.br/index.php/psicanalise- baroque/article/download/7384/6517 . Accessed July 15, 2018.

SOUZA, Alexandre Candido de; MELO, Claudia Virginia de Brito. **The Brazilian labor market in the face of an aging population**. In: Brasil 2050 [electronic resource] : desafios de uma nagao que envelhecer / Camara dos Deputados, Centro de Estudos e Debates Estrategicos, Consultoria Legislativa; rapporteur Cristiane Brasil; legislative consultants Alexandre Candido de Souza (coord.), Alberto Pinheiro [et al.]. - Brasilia : Camara dos Deputados, Edigoes Camara, 2017. - (Serie estudos estrategicos; n. 8 PDF).

SOUZA, J. L. C. **Asylum for the elderly: the place of the rejected face.** Jornal da Universidade Federal do Para, Belem, year 4, n° 1, p. 2, 2003.

SOUZA. Noelma Cavalcante; MENEZES, Antonio Basilio Novaes Thomaz de Meneses. **Disciplinary power: a reading in Surveillance and Punishment.** In: Saberes, Natal - RN, v. 1, n.4, jun 2010. Available: https://periodicos.ufrn.br/saberes/article/viewFile/561/510 . Accessed July 12, 2018.

TEIXEIRA, Solange. **Social policies in Brazil: the history (and current) relationship between the "public" and the "private" in the Brazilian social protection system**. In: Sociedade em debate, Pelotas, 13(2), 45-64. Jun-Dec, 2007. Available at: http://www.revistas.ucpel.tche.br/index.php/rsd/article/viewFile/400/354. Accessed on June 30, 2018.

TOREZAN. Z. C. F. and AGUIAR. F. **The subject of psychoanalysis: particularity**

in contemporaneity. Revista Mal Estar e Subjetividade. vol.11 no.2 Fortaleza 2011.

VERAS, Renato. **Pals jovem com cabelos brancos: a saude do idoso no Brasil.** Rio de Janeiro: Relume Dumara/UERJ, 1994

WANZELER, Murilo Cunha. **Self-care in Michel Foucault.** Master's thesis - UFRB/CCHLA. Supervisor: Paulo Tarso Cabral Medeiros. 2011. Available at: http://tede.biblioteca.ufpb.br/bitstream/tede/5579/1/arquivototal.pdf. Accessed on July 09, 2018.

WORLD HEALTH ORGANIZATION. **Active ageing: a health policy"** / World Health Organization. Brasilia: Pan American Health Organization, 2005. Available at: http://bvsms.saude.gov.br/bvs/publicacoes/envelhecimento_ativo.pdf. Accessed on July 11, 2018.

APPENDIX

Product of the dissertation:

TRAINING SEMINAR FOR MANAGERS AND PROFESSIONALS OF ILPI'S.

THE INTERFACE BETWEEN GERONTOLOGY AND CARE PRACTICES.

This seminar is part of the positions developed by the master's student around the analysis and contextualization of the Long Stay Institutions for the Elderly - ILPI's supported by the public policies in force in Brazil.

Target audience: Professionals and managers who work in ILPI's.

Seminar to train managers and professionals from ILPI's - The interface between gerontology and care practices.

Objective: To establish a permanent dialog between nursing homes and society, in order to guarantee a new democratic and innovative practice in the care processes for the elderly living in ILPIs.

Date: September 28, 2018

Hours: 8:00 a.m. to 5:00 p.m.

Address: Public Ministry of the State of Rio de Janeiro

Av. Marechal Camara, n° 370 / 9° andar, Centro - Rio de Janeiro

Registration: www.unatiuerj.com.br

Programming:

8:00 am - Opening

Dr[3] . Cristiane Branquinho Lucas

(Coordinator of the Operational Support Center for People with Disabilities and the Elderly)

- Public Ministry of Rio de Janeiro)

Sandra Rabello de Frias

(Coordinator of UNATI / UERJ Extension Projects)

9 a.m. to 9:40 a.m. - Personnel Management and Administration of LTCFs

9h50 to 10h30 - The Importance of Valuing Care

10h40 to 11h20 - The Approach to the Demented Elderly

11:30 a.m. to 12:10 p.m. - The Importance of Interdisciplinary Care in LTCFs

13h to 14h - Break and lunch

14h30 to 16h30 - Simultaneous workshops

- MPRJ's roadmap for inspecting ILPIs
- Accessibility / fall prevention
- Nutrition in LTCFs 16h30 to 17h - Proposals Forum and Closing Ceremony

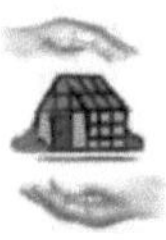

Seminário de capacitação de gestores e profissionais de ILPI's – A interface da gerontologia junto às práticas de cuidado.

TEMA: A IMPORTÂNCIA DA INTERDISCIPLINARIDADE DO CUIDADO NAS ILPI's

LOCAL: AUDITÓRIO DO MINISTÉRIO PÚBLICO
Av. Marechal Camara, 370/9º andar

DATA: 28 de Setembro de 2018

HORÁRIO: 8:00 horas às 17:00 horas

TRAINING SEMINAR FOR MANAGERS AND PROFESSIONALS OF ILPI'S.

THE INTERFACE BETWEEN GERONTOLOGY AND CARE PRACTICES.

REGISTRATION FORM

Name:

Address:

N°:____________Bairro:__________________________CEP:____________________

Telefone (s):________________________________/___________________________

E-mail:

____

Professional Training: ( ) YES ( ) NO

Which one?

____

Do you specialize in Geriatrics or Gerontology? ( ) YES ( ) NO

Which one?

____

Have you taken any courses in caring for the elderly? ( ) YES ( ) NO

Which one?

____

Which institution do you work for?

____

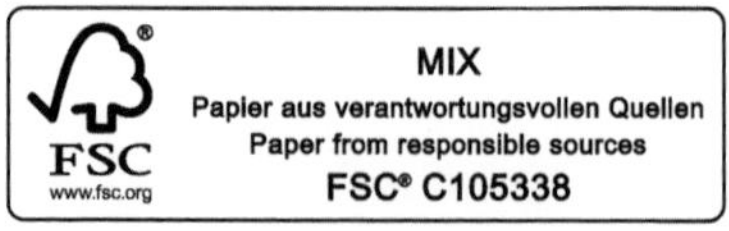

Printed by Books on Demand GmbH, Norderstedt / Germany